I0800497

IMAGES
of America

DIXMONT STATE HOSPITAL

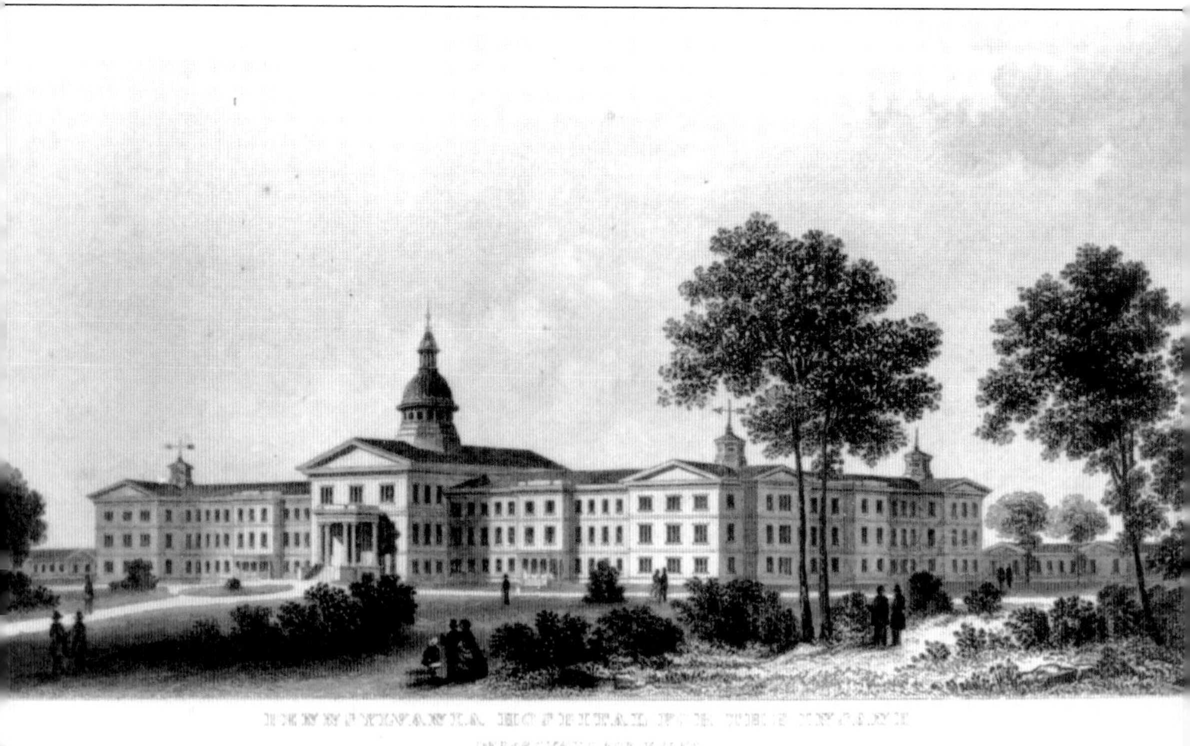

The idea to build Dixmont stemmed from the overcrowding of the Western Pennsylvania Hospital's insane department, which, by 1855, had sprawled into other departments of the hospital. The managers of the Western Pennsylvania Hospital turned no one away as long as there was space for an additional cot. This philosophy, however, led to overcrowding and conditions that were not acceptable for a hospital environment. By May 1, 1859, construction on Dixmont had begun based on the Thomas Kirkbride design utilized in the Pennsylvania Hospital for the Insane in Philadelphia. The design was adopted by many hospitals nationwide.

On the cover: Reed Hall, named after Dixmont's first superintendent, Dr. Joseph Allison Reed, was the main administrative building of the hospital. The building is based upon architecture conceived by Thomas Kirkbride. Photographs of Reed Hall and the hospital grounds were frequently included in the annual manager's reports for the hospital. (Courtesy Ben Avon Area Historical Association.)

IMAGES
of America

DIXMONT STATE HOSPITAL

Mark Berton

ARCADIA
PUBLISHING

ISBN 978-0-7385-4520-2

Published by Arcadia Publishing
Charleston, South Carolina

Printed in the United States of America

Library of Congress Catalog Card Number: 2006922345

For all general information contact Arcadia Publishing at:
Telephone 843-853-2070
Fax 843-853-0044
E-mail sales@arcadiapublishing.com
For customer service and orders:
Toll-Free 1-888-313-2665

Visit us on the Internet at www.arcadiapublishing.com

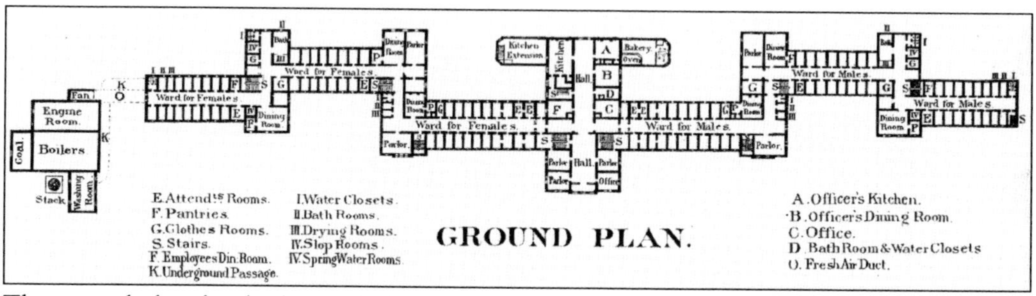

The ground plan for the hospital, depicted here, shows the northern wing of Reed Hall (left side) housed females, while the southern wing was devoted to males. Administrative offices and food preparation areas were in the center of the hospital. This bat wing–like architecture was conceived by Thomas Kirkbride and allowed hospital officials to add wards as needed without disturbing existing wards. On November 13, 1862, 113 patients were transferred to Dixmont.

CONTENTS

ACKNOWLEDGMENTS

This book is the product of a fascination that began one hot day in July 1999, when I first signed off on the waiver of liability for the Stroyne Family Limited Partnership, giving me permission to set foot on the 407 acres that were Dixmont State Hospital.

It was humid and sticky, what one would expect as normal for Pittsburgh in July. But what struck me as odd was the fact that there were no birds or insects rustling the thick brush that grew up around Dixmont's main building, Reed Hall. At that point, my reason gave way to imagination, and it was perhaps the only time that I felt intimidated by the enormous structure and its outlying buildings.

Since then, I have met with ghost hunters, urban explorers, photographers, psychics, former employees, neighbors, and more. Many people have fallen prey to the allure of the imaginative aspects of an abandoned asylum. But, for having spent hundreds of hours walking the halls of the buildings that made up Dixmont, I can honestly say Dixmont is more fascinating for what it is––a piece of history—than what it is not––a haunted house.

The ghosts that wander the halls of Dixmont are historical ghosts, former doctors, nurses, and patients who all have contributed to the cause of mental health care. These are friendly ghosts who have revealed to me an institution dedicated to the humane treatment of the mentally ill. Yes, the details of mental health care can be gruesome and misunderstood. Yes, treatments can seem barbaric to the uninitiated. However, what aspect of past medical practices does not seem barbaric or extreme by today's standards?

This book is a pictorial rendition of the living Dixmont, the hospital that served thousands of mentally ill patients in western Pennsylvania. I hope to present to you a beautiful and complex institution, built on ground chosen by Dorothea Lynde Dix herself for its pastoral and relaxing quality.

Since that first day in 1999, I have explored and photographed many other mental institutions in the region––Norristown, Torrance, Woodville, Mayview, Pilgrim State, and more. None of those excursions can compare to the full access and freedom that was granted me at Dixmont. I thank the Stroyne family––Ralph, Tim, and Carol—for supporting my curiosity and giving me such a unique insight into such a wonderful world. I also would like to thank Tony Chammas of ASC Development, Christine Davis of Christine Davis Consultants, Tracy Ferguson, Barry Chad, Beth Cummins, Helen Wolf, Leroy Egan, Jack Lennon, Tom Patton, Robert Grom, and all those I have met along the way who have helped out in filling in the holes of Dixmont's past.

I dedicate this book to my parents, Joann Berton and Robert Burns.

INTRODUCTION

At a time when many historic psychiatric institutions are facing closure and demolition, when towns and cities are reconsidering the uses of such land, and when psychiatry has significantly evolved from the initial intentions that inspired their founding, historians around the country struggle to document the history of these vast structures and the stories of those who had been there. In retrospect, we can now begin to see how their course was influenced by inner and outer circumstances alike, taking turns and detours over the decades that none of the founders could have foreseen.

Dixmont State Hospital is 1 of 60 historic institutions built nationwide with a particular symmetrical design, the Kirkbride plan, and within a particular time frame, 1850–1883. But among these 60 Kirkbride hospitals, Dixmont stands out as the one that is most reminiscent of the legendary Dorothea Lynde Dix, whose reform-driven efforts at establishing asylums for the mentally ill in dozens of states were both astonishing and unparalleled. It was Miss Dix in her gray dress, always in transit, always negotiating with state legislators, who insisted that Dixmont would not be placed in the heart of Pittsburgh, but that, instead, it would be built outside of the city, surrounded by nature. She described the hilltop setting she had chosen for Dixmont as "both salubrious and cheerful, joined with outlooks of rare beauty associated with some elements of grandeur." And the place was indeed all of that, as can be seen from the old photographs. Facing west and overlooking the Ohio River, its setting was gorgeous without sacrificing function and practicality. Studying the plans and early images of Dixmont, we marvel at the details of the architecture, its decorations, and the landscaping. Much of the decor was lost over time, but the strange, majestic appeal of the grand old brick buildings overlooking the valley remained unchanged until their demolition in 2006.

As we sort through this history, we have to remember that state hospitals were more than mere sites of a specific architecture. Oftentimes they served as a last refuge to those who had nowhere else to go, no other option to find treatment and help for a mental illness. Equally as often, they became places of isolation and confinement, neglect and abuse. Hospital employees are known for saying that they had to "make do with less than nothing" and that they "did the best they could" when facing recurrent shortages of funding, personnel, medication, and space. Many of the old state hospitals never received the funds that were needed to take care of their patients in an appropriate way, let alone make renovations and investments in the architecture. And thus, the crumbling of these places began long before their closings.

Perhaps now it becomes clear that the 19th-century vision of Dixmont's founders was too closely linked to a rigid type of architecture that would not be flexible enough to face the enormous medical and social challenges of the 20th century. It proved impossible to continue operations on the original grand, peaceful, and benevolent scale. In the face of creating less restrictive psychiatric settings and seeking reintegration of patients into the community, Dixmont had become an inheritance from the past, difficult to find modern use for. With its demolition, Dixmont's remarkable history is now closed, and we turn to archives, books, and oral histories to allow us back in and discover what life in one of the country's premier state hospitals was like. So many lives were touched by this hospital, so many memories shaped.

—Anna Schuleit, June 2006

One

Reform and Build

The story of Dixmont could have been very different were it not for its namesake, Dorothea Lynde Dix. The desire to build a hospital for the mentally ill of western Pennsylvania stemmed from the overcrowding of the newly opened Western Pennsylvania Hospital in Pittsburgh. That hospital's capacity was 100 patients and 20 mental patients. By 1854, the hospital admitted 172 patients, and the need for relief was apparent. The insane department had taken over most of the hospital's resources. The hospital's board of directors entertained two alternatives: build a new wing or build a new hospital. Dix, whose interest in mental health care reform brought her to Pittsburgh, advocated for a completely new facility for the insane department, then run by Dr. Joseph Allison Reed. The initial site for the hospital was Homestead, on a property later occupied by the Edgar Thompson Steel Works. The property was purchased then sold when Dix disapproved of the location. Vowing to find a new location, Dix found a more suitable site upon a plateau overlooking the Ohio River. Her name was forever bound to the site in 1860 when Western Pennsylvania Hospital president Thomas Bakewell named the railroad station serving the site Dixmont.

Intended to serve 21 counties in western Pennsylvania, construction began on the Western Pennsylvania Hospital for the Insane at Dixmont in May 1859. By 1862, the entire structure was completed, and 113 patients were transferred to the 585-bed facility. Only two patients remained at Western Pennsylvania; neither was mentally ill.

The hospital received its own charter and a name change to the Dixmont Hospital for the Insane in 1907. The name was shortened to the Dixmont Hospital in 1921 after managers filed a petition with the courts to change the name of the corporation specifically to remove the wording "for the Insane."

The institution was partially a state corporation because the governor of Pennsylvania appointed members to the board of directors and the state funded part of the hospital's operation. The last name change came in 1945, when ownership of Dixmont was transferred to the State of Pennsylvania by state statute, creating Dixmont State Hospital.

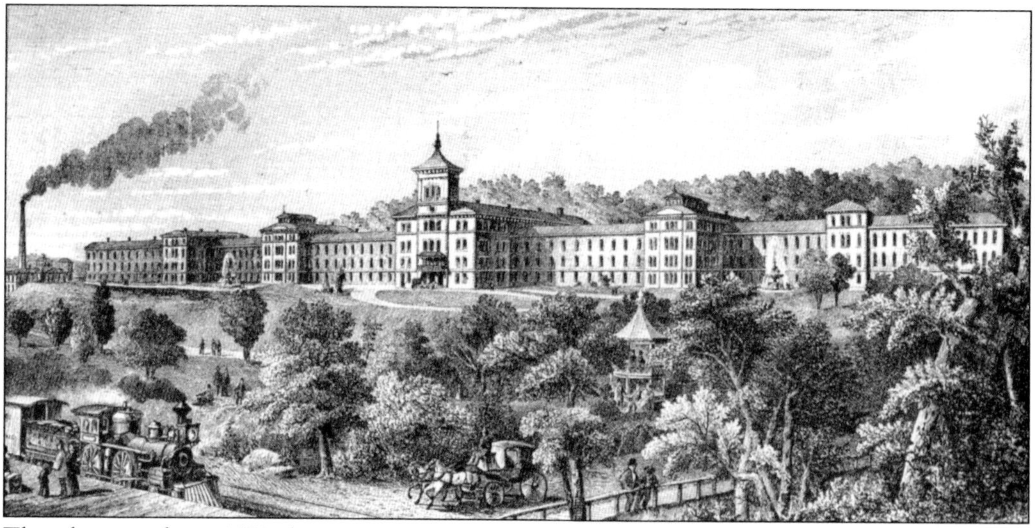

This drawing from 1870 shows Dixmont and incorporates all of the attributes to make the site viable for a mental health care facility—railroad, roadway, lush vegetation, and gorgeous architecture. However, the proximity of these attributes is not to scale in this representation. Dixmont sat on more than 400 acres of property.

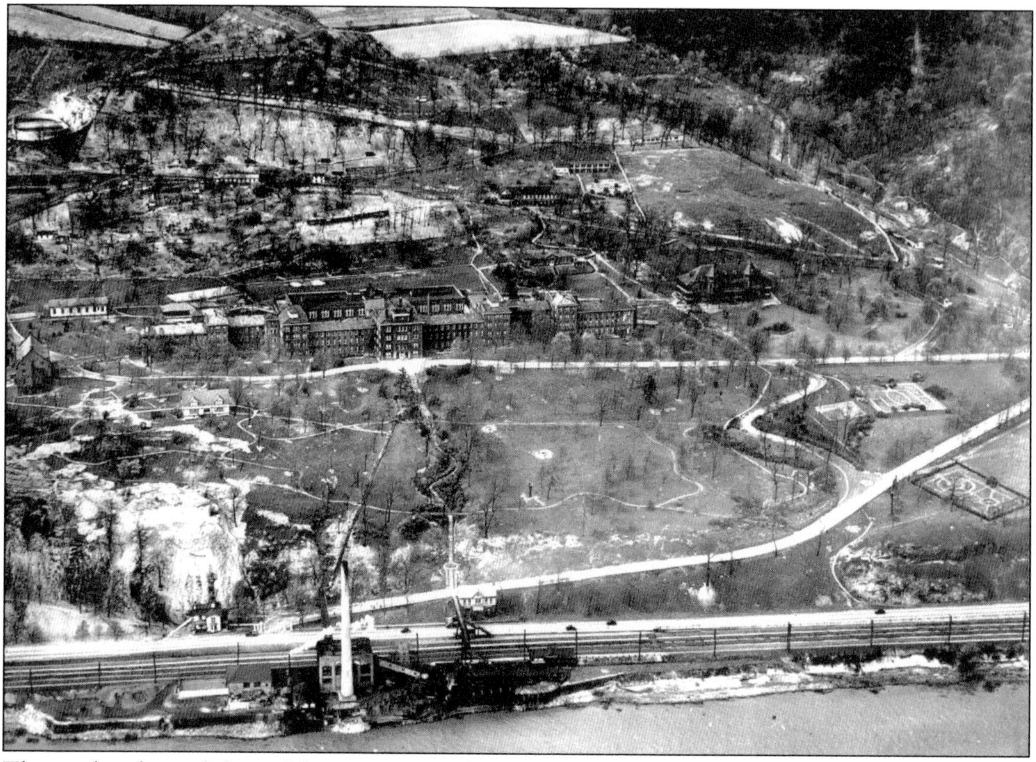

This undated aerial shot of the majority of the Dixmont property clearly shows how the hospital had everything on site to be its own self-sufficient community. The boiler house is along the train tracks at the bottom of the image. Reed Hall is in the center of the photograph, and the reservoir is in the upper left quadrant. Other buildings easily seen in this photograph include the men's annex, post office, and train station.

William Anderson Herron, pictured here, was a member of Western Pennsylvania Hospital's board of directors and later a member of Dixmont's executive committee. Herron was a highly influential Pittsburgher who devoted himself to the advancement of charitable causes. Not only holding high positions at Dixmont and Western Pennsylvania Hospitals, he also was vice president of both the Blind Asylum of Western Pennsylvania and the Homeopathic Hospital.

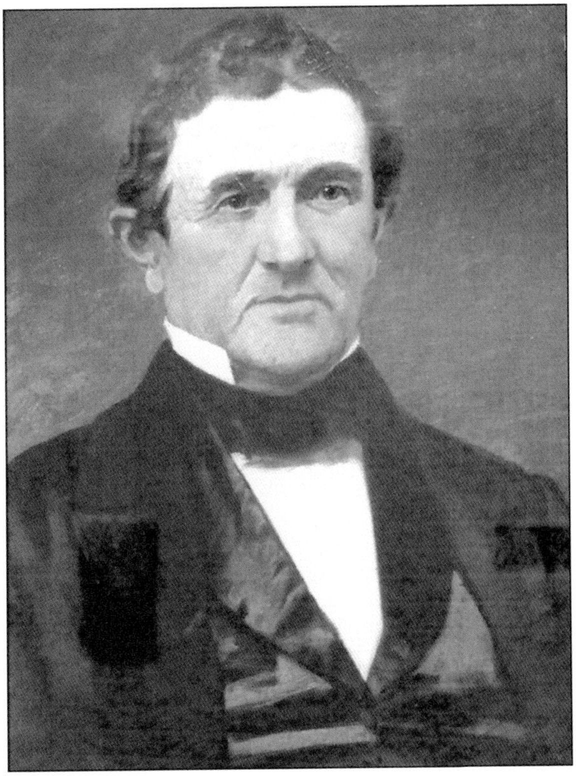

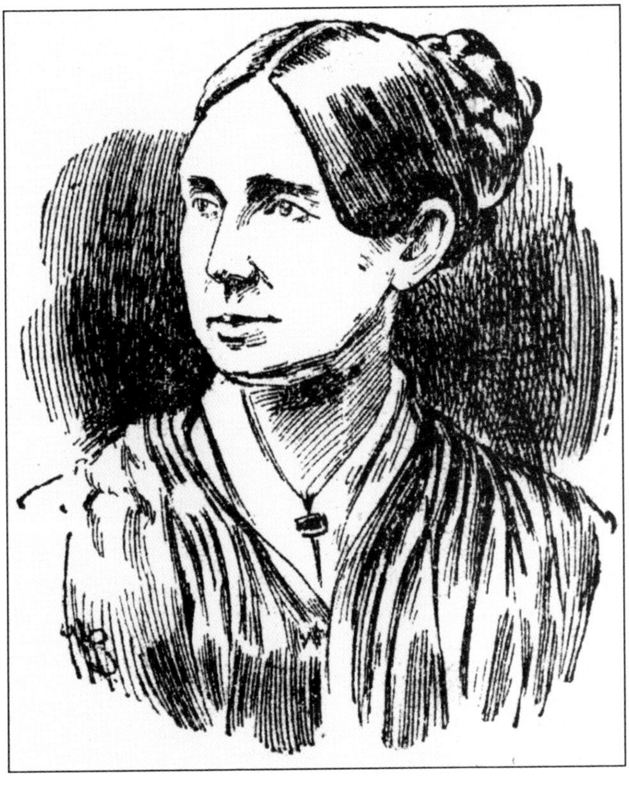

Famous for her role in mental health care reform, Dorothea Lynde Dix was instrumental in choosing the site of the Western Pennsylvania Hospital for the Insane at Dixmont. Her name became attached to the hospital officially in 1860 when the Western Pennsylvania Hospital Board of Directors named the train station that served the hospital Dixmont.

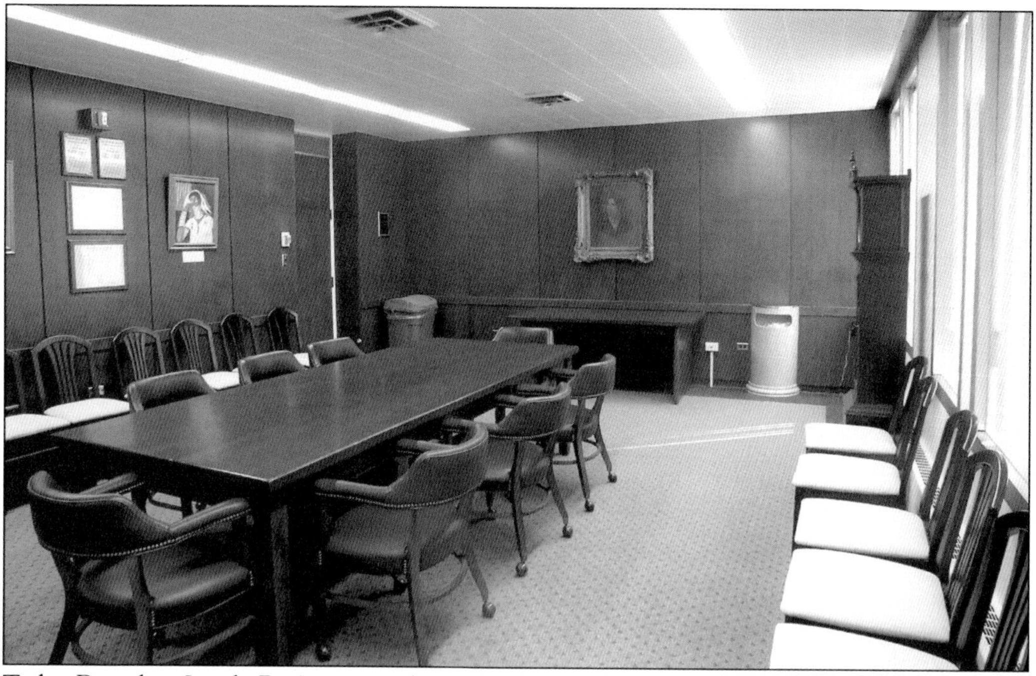

Today Dorothea Lynde Dix's portrait hangs in the conference room inside the Bengs Building at Mayview State Hospital. When Dixmont closed in 1984, antiques and artifacts from the hospital's past were transferred to Mayview State Hospital, where they remain. The portrait was given to the hospital by an anonymous donor in 1865. It hung in Dixmont's conference room while the hospital was open. (Courtesy www.dixmontstate.com.)

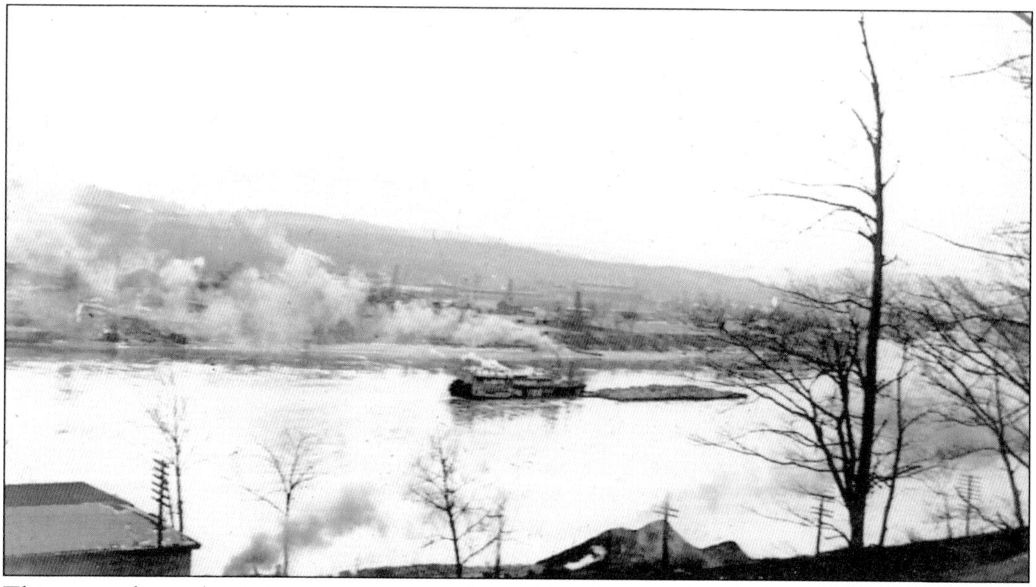

This view from the Dixmont property shows Neville Island, which was fertile farmland, particularly known for its strawberry fields, when Dixmont was built. Over time, Neville Island transformed into an industrial site, home to chemical plants and factories. The island, once called Montour Island, was named after Gen. John Neville. It was given to Neville by Congress in observance of his military service in the Revolutionary War.

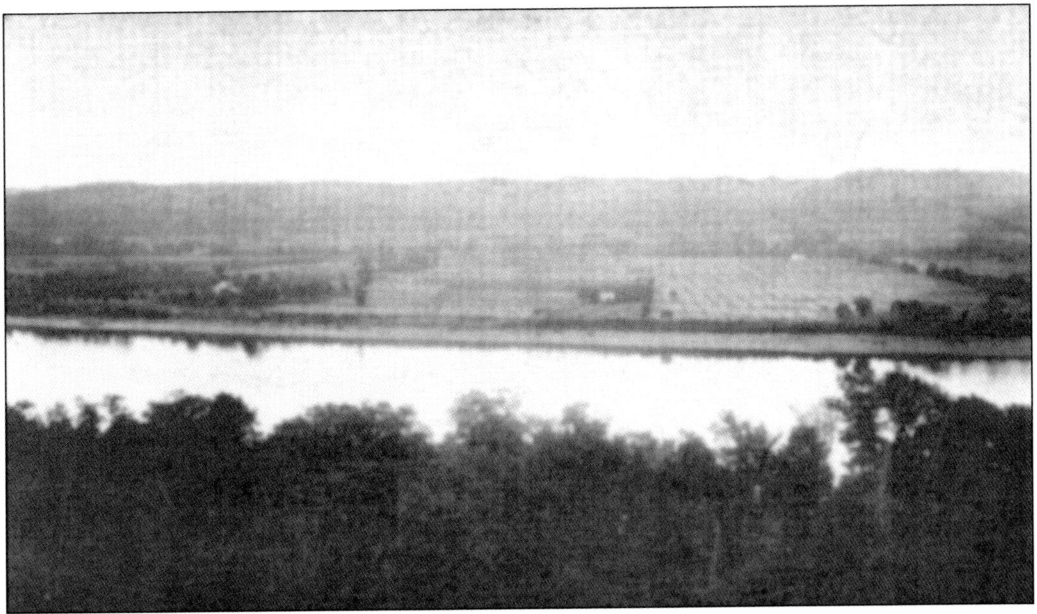

Another view from Dixmont shows the vast overlook of the surrounding areas that Dixmont had. In his history of Dixmont, published in internal staff newsletters over several years, Dr. Anibal Herrera wrote, "The location of the buildings on a plateau sufficiently situated to offer a view of several miles of the Ohio River and unsurpassed facilities for drainage, and through ventilation of the buildings by natural and artificial means."

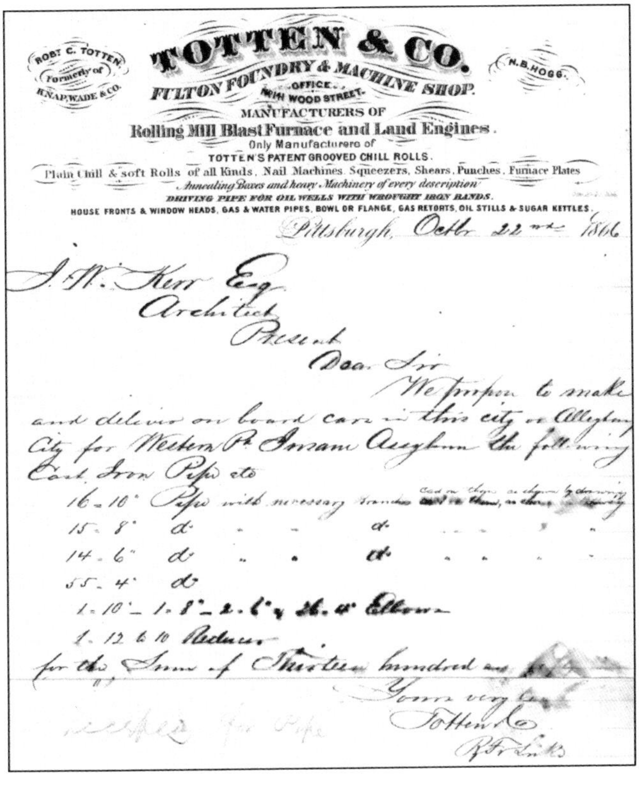

ROBT C. TOTTEN, Formerly of KNAP, WADE & CO.

TOTTEN & CO.

N. B. HOGG.

FULTON FOUNDRY & MACHINE SHOP.

OFFICE, 141 WOOD STREET.

MANUFACTURERS OF

Rolling Mill Blast Furnace and Land Engines.

Only Manufacturers of

TOTTEN'S PATENT GROOVED CHILL ROLLS.

Plain Chill & soft Rolls of all Kinds, Nail Machines, Squeezers, Shears, Punches, Furnace Plates

Annealing Boxes and heavy Machinery of every description

DRIVING PIPE FOR OIL WELLS WITH WROUGHT IRON BANDS.

HOUSE FRONTS & WINDOW HEADS, GAS & WATER PIPES, BOWL OR FLANGE, GAS RETORTS, OIL STILLS & SUGAR KETTLES.

Pittsburgh, Octbr 22nd 1866

J. W. Kerr Esq.
Architect
Present
Dear Sir
We propose to make and deliver on board cars in this city or Allegheny City for Western Pa Insane Asylum the following Cast Iron Pipe etc

The board of directors for the Western Pennsylvania Hospital commissioned architect J. R. Kerr to design Dixmont. Kerr was extremely involved in every detail of Dixmont's construction. This invoice dated October 22, 1866, is for various lengths of pipe from the Totten and Company Machine Shop. What is notable about this invoice is that it states at the top that J. R. Kerr, Dixmont's architect, was present at the signing. It also refers to Allegheny City, which was absorbed by a growing Pittsburgh in 1907. Other invoices detail minutiae such as the dimensions of the brick to be used for the building. The entire design of the building was based on Thomas Kirkbride's basic design for mental health facilities, which is known by sweeping batlike wings and symmetry. (Courtesy the Stroyne family collection.)

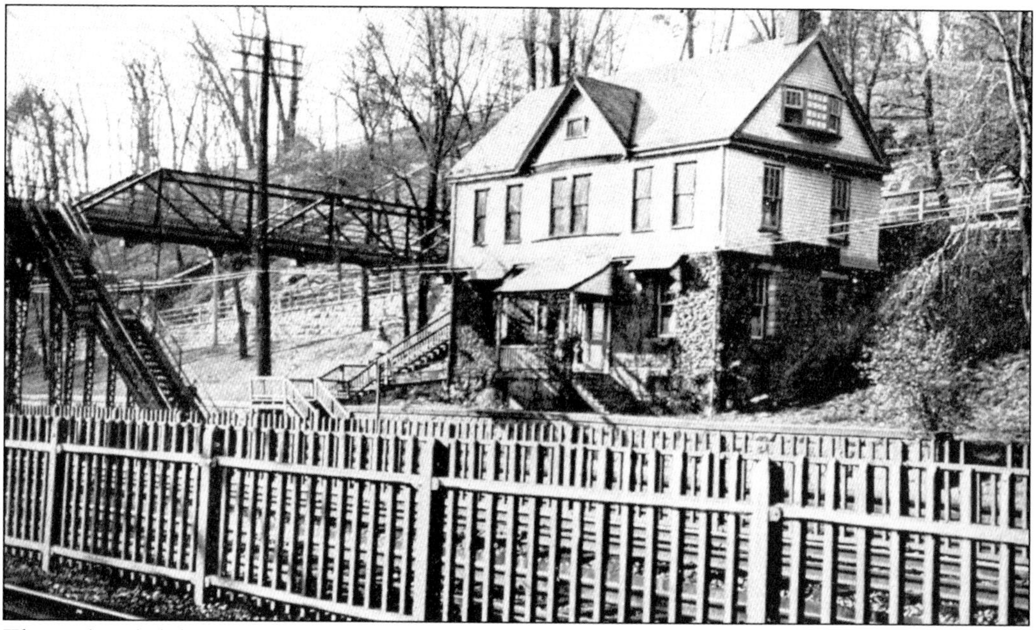

The railroad did not only connect Dixmont to the city of Pittsburgh. Several miles up the Ohio River, it served the population of Sewickley. Sewickley was a bedroom community for rich industrialists desiring to get out of the then smoggy and sooty conditions of downtown Pittsburgh. Today the railroad tracks still run adjacent to the Dixmont property and Route 65.

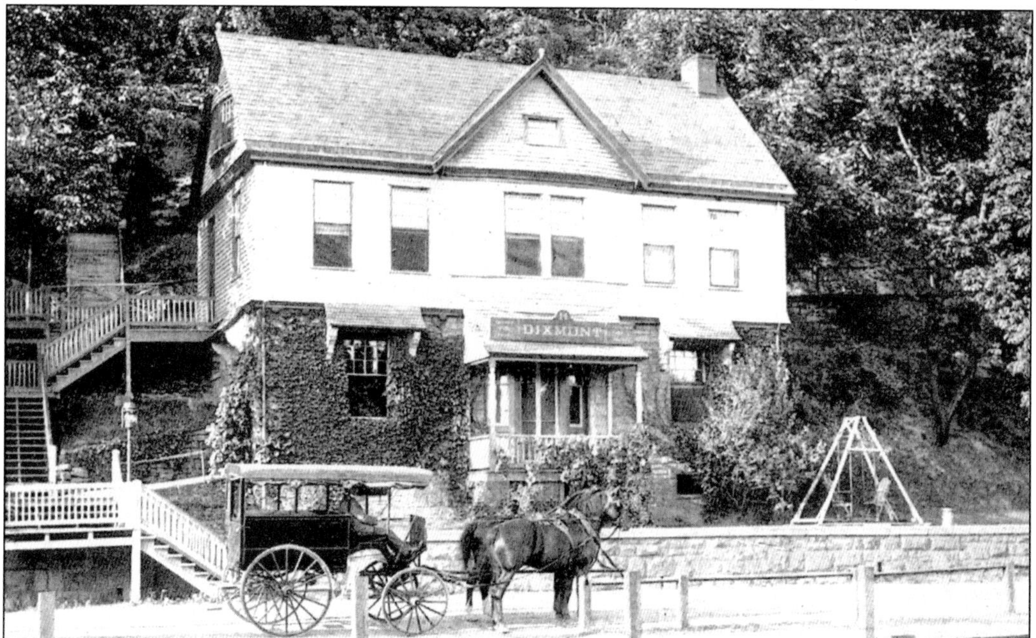

Dixmont had its own post office, shown here in the year 1900. The post office was on what was then called Beaver Plank Road, but is Route 65 today. The postmaster and family lived in the second-floor apartment thanks to an addition to the building made in 1877. The structure also housed the ticket agent for the railroad. It was ordered to be vacated by January 1, 1954, in preparation for the widening of Route 65.

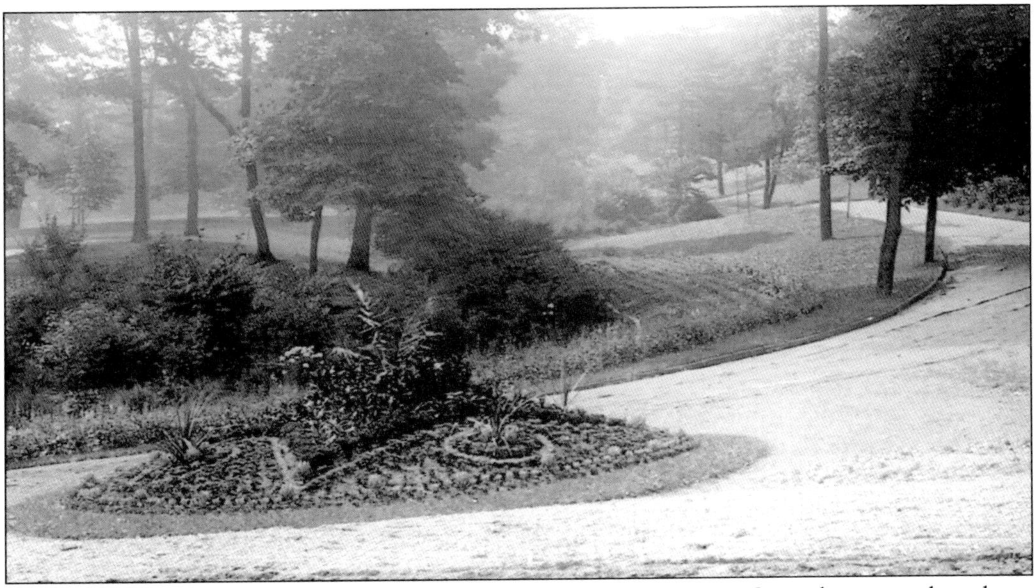

This *c.* 1915 postcard shows one of the roads on Dixmont's campus. Over the years, there have been many roads and driveways cut through the property. When the hospital closed in 1984, the main road started at Huntington Avenue and cut fairly straight through the property to Toms Run Road on the opposite side. While the Toms Run side was supposed to be a delivery entrance, records from the mid-1960s show that most traffic came to the hospital through the residential Huntington Avenue entrance, angering neighbors. (Courtesy of the Stroyne Family Collection.)

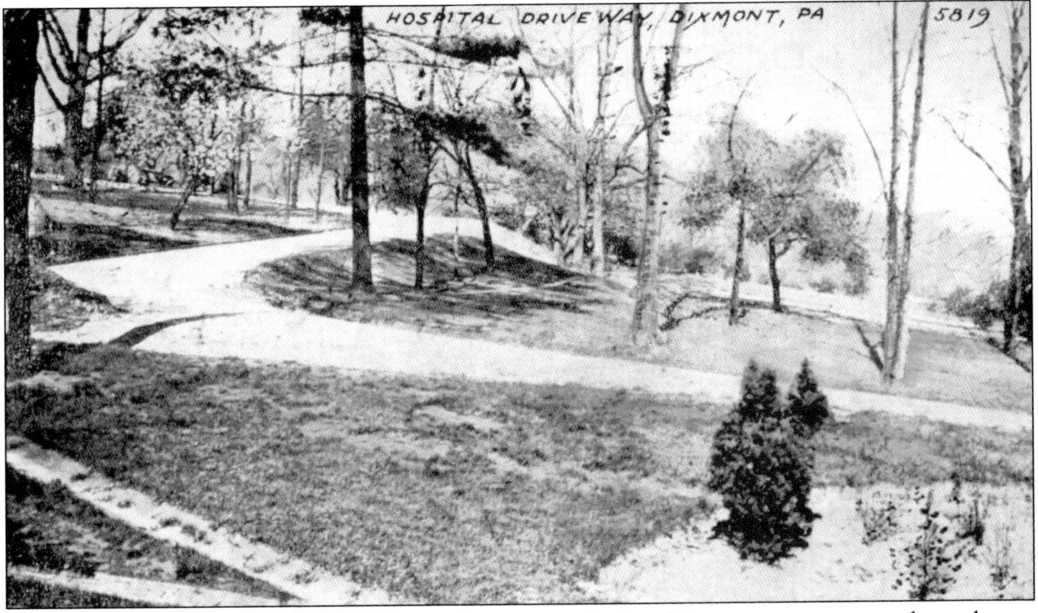

This undated postcard shows yet another view of the Dixmont campus and roadways. Superintendent Henry Hutchinson wrote in an annual report for 1934 that patients who were offered the opportunity to work usually preferred to work outside on the lawns, driveways, and grounds: "a large number were engaged throughout the year in the greenhouse and in the industrial departments." (Courtesy the Stroyne family collection.)

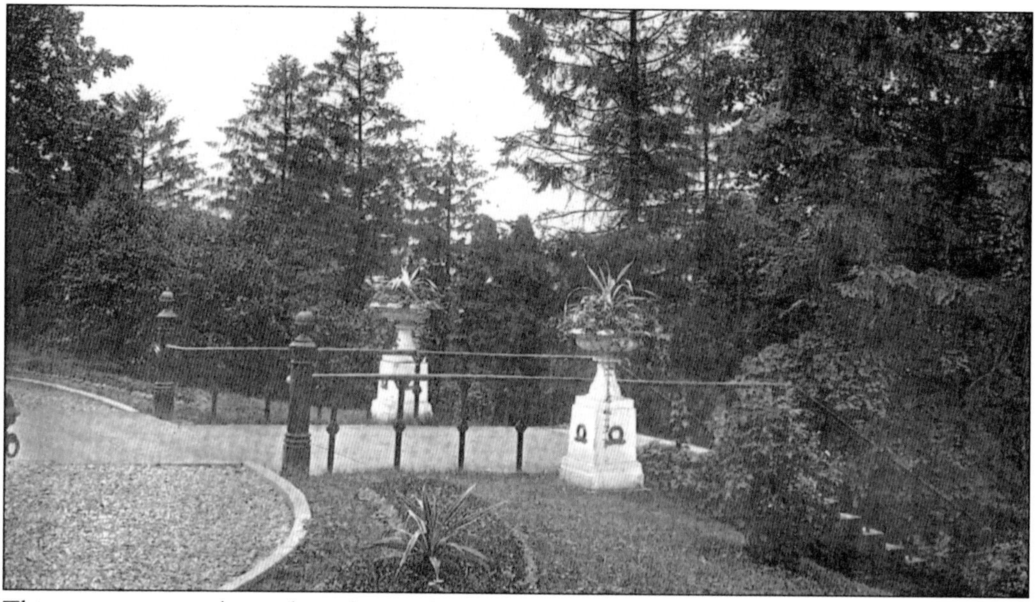

This stairway was located in front of Reed Hall and is flanked by two decorative urns. Beautification of the grounds was an ongoing pursuit of Dr. Joseph Allison Reed. Much of this work was completed without state funding, using paying patients and benefactors as funding sources. The overall plan for grounds beautification was conceived by Donald. G. Mitchell, a well-known artist of the time.

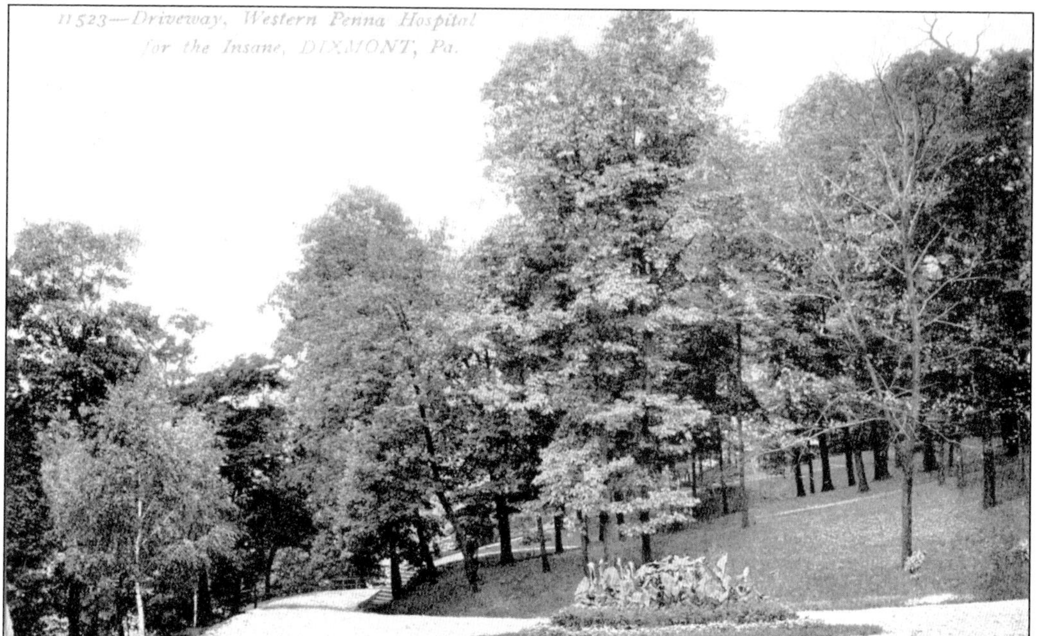
11523—Driveway, Western Penna Hospital
for the Insane, DIXMONT, Pa.

This postcard shows the driveway of Dixmont. Even though there were many roads and throughways crisscrossing the property, the site did not have official street names until 1971 when, under the superintendence of Dr. Robert Weimer, a contest was held to name the roads on the property. Once decided, road signs were ordered from the state and erected. (Courtesy the Stroyne family collection.)

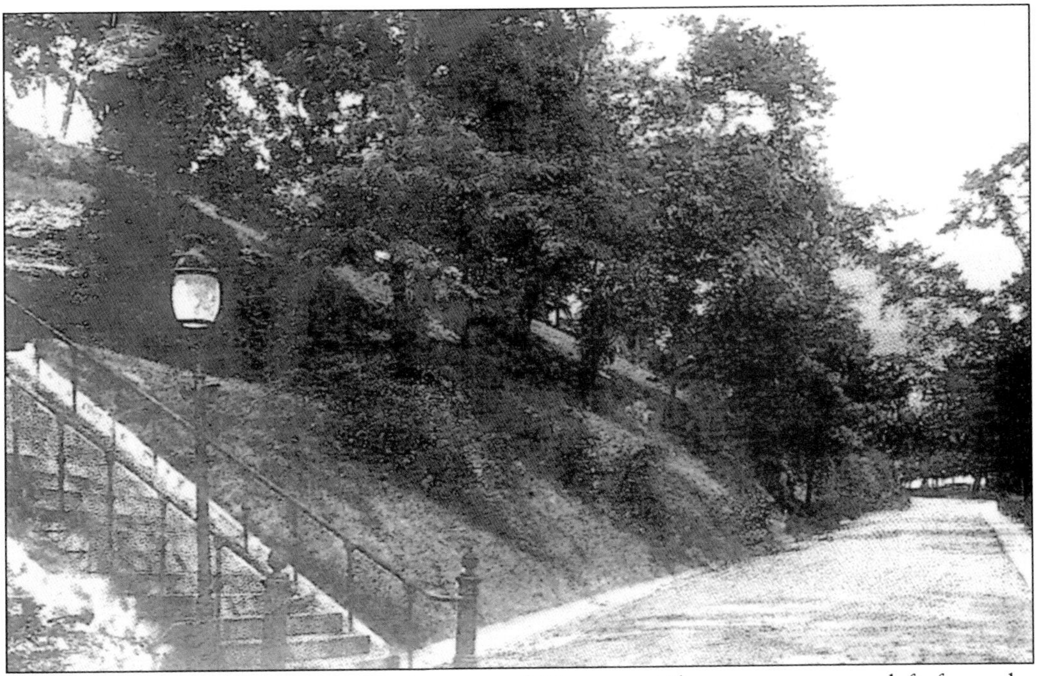

This photograph shows the main driveway of Dixmont. The entrance was cleft from the property during a road-widening project along old Beaver Plank Road, now Route 65. The project converted the road from a two-lane road to a four-lane divided highway and required the removal of tons of rock from the base of the hill abutting Dixmont's property.

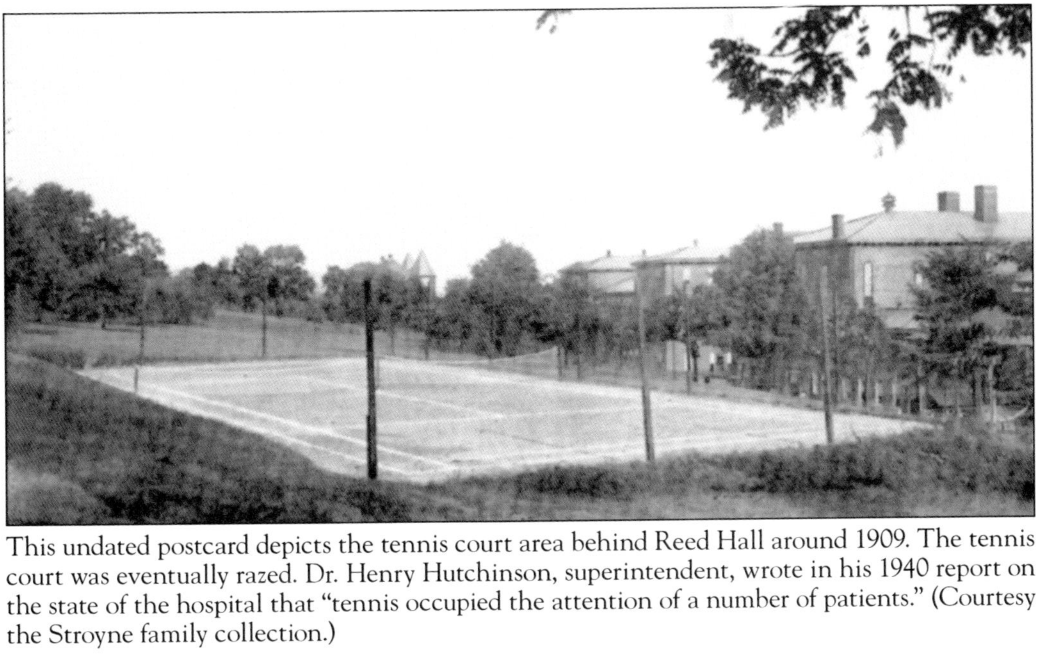

This undated postcard depicts the tennis court area behind Reed Hall around 1909. The tennis court was eventually razed. Dr. Henry Hutchinson, superintendent, wrote in his 1940 report on the state of the hospital that "tennis occupied the attention of a number of patients." (Courtesy the Stroyne family collection.)

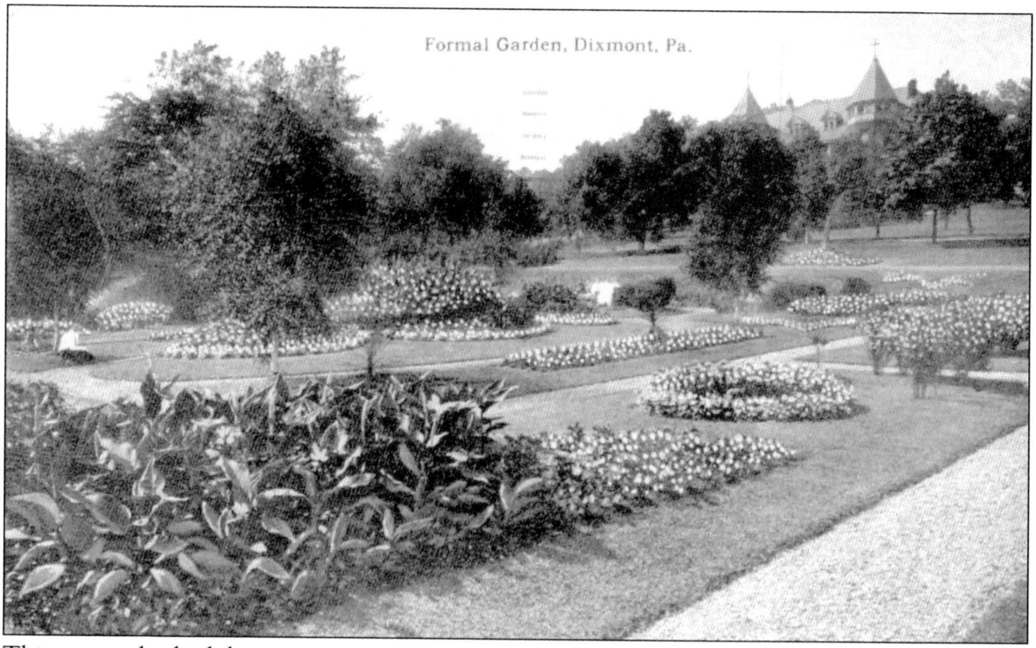

This postcard, which has a stamp cancellation of April 8, 1914, depicts the glorious Victorian-style gardens that once flourished at Dixmont. The distinctive architecture of the men's annex building can clearly be seen in the background. In the center, several nurses can be seen sitting on a bench. The hand-written message on the back of the postcard reads simply, "Dear Dad, All O.K. Freddie." (Courtesy the Stroyne family collection.)

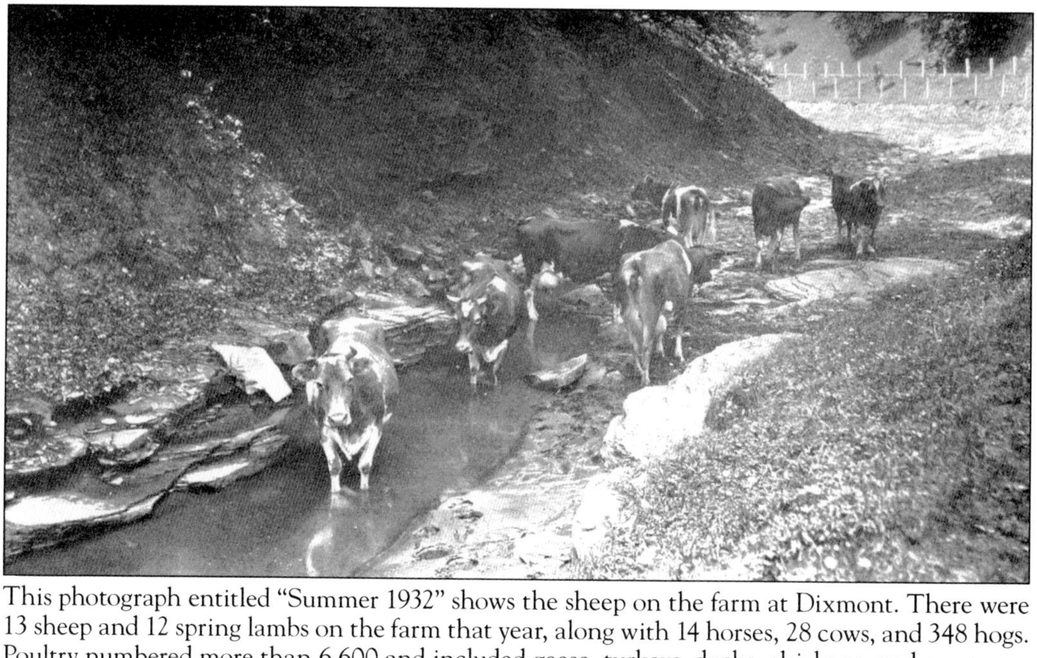

This photograph entitled "Summer 1932" shows the sheep on the farm at Dixmont. There were 13 sheep and 12 spring lambs on the farm that year, along with 14 horses, 28 cows, and 348 hogs. Poultry numbered more than 6,600 and included geese, turkeys, ducks, chickens, and roosters.

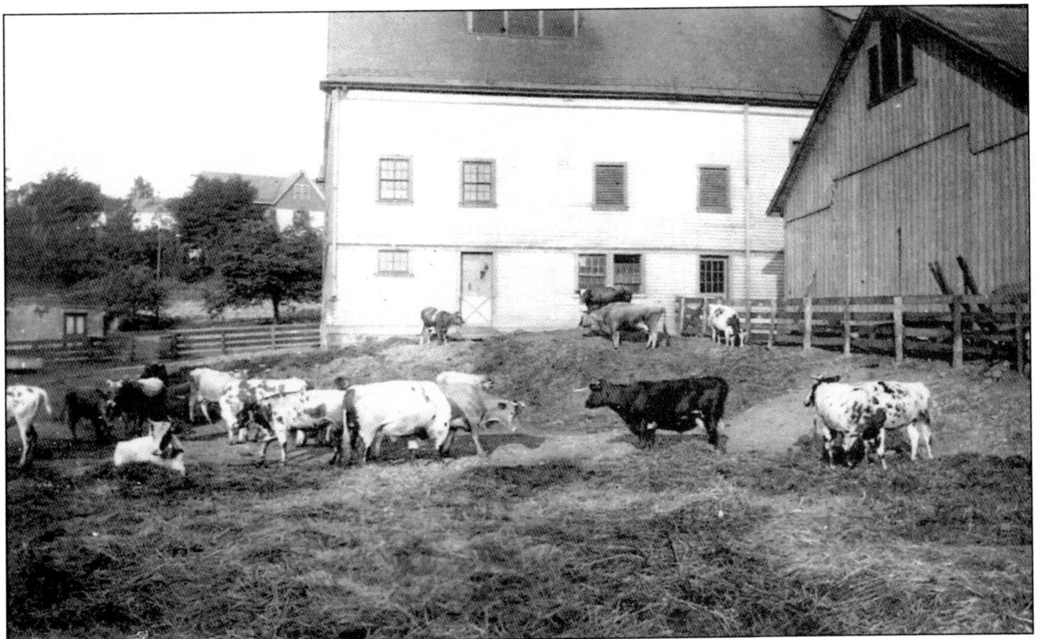

The Dixmont property was comprised of more than 400 acres formed from the purchase and consolidation of the Backhouse, Ryan, and Gilliland farms. As Dixmont evolved, it continued its tradition of agricultural pursuits. Shown here is a dairy barn and cows on the Dixmont property. Many of the agricultural duties were performed by recovering patients, as well as staff. In 1869, approximately six acres were set aside for crops, and farming was an activity encouraged by Dr. Joseph Allison Reed.

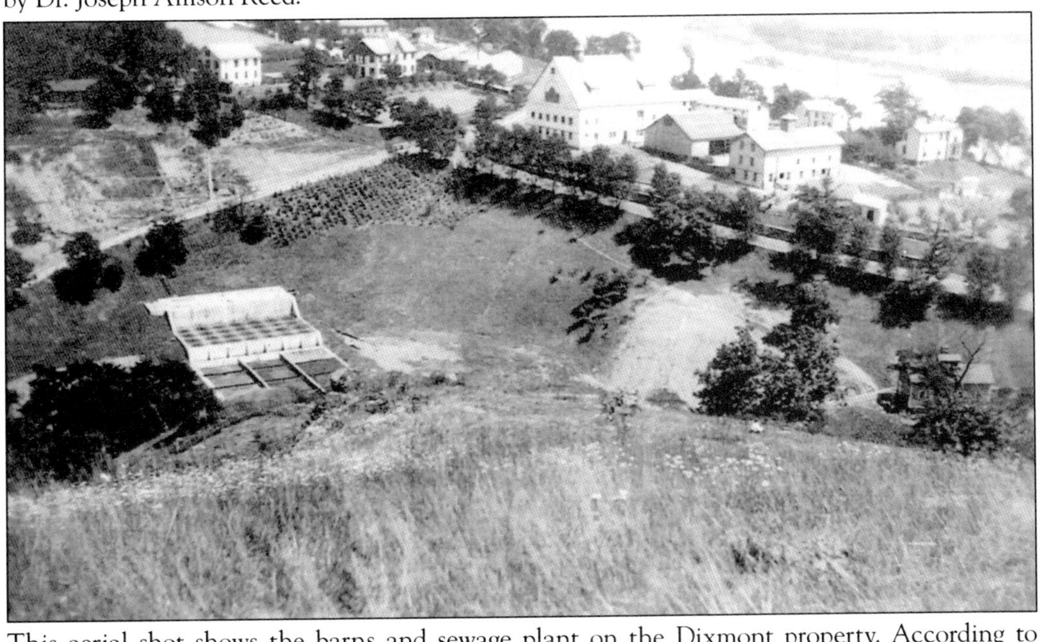

This aerial shot shows the barns and sewage plant on the Dixmont property. According to archeological studies, Dixmont had more than 80 buildings at one time, including several barns, a farmhouse, a stable, and a piggery that could accommodate up to 40 Berkshire hogs. The piggery was discontinued in 1956 and demolished in 1962.

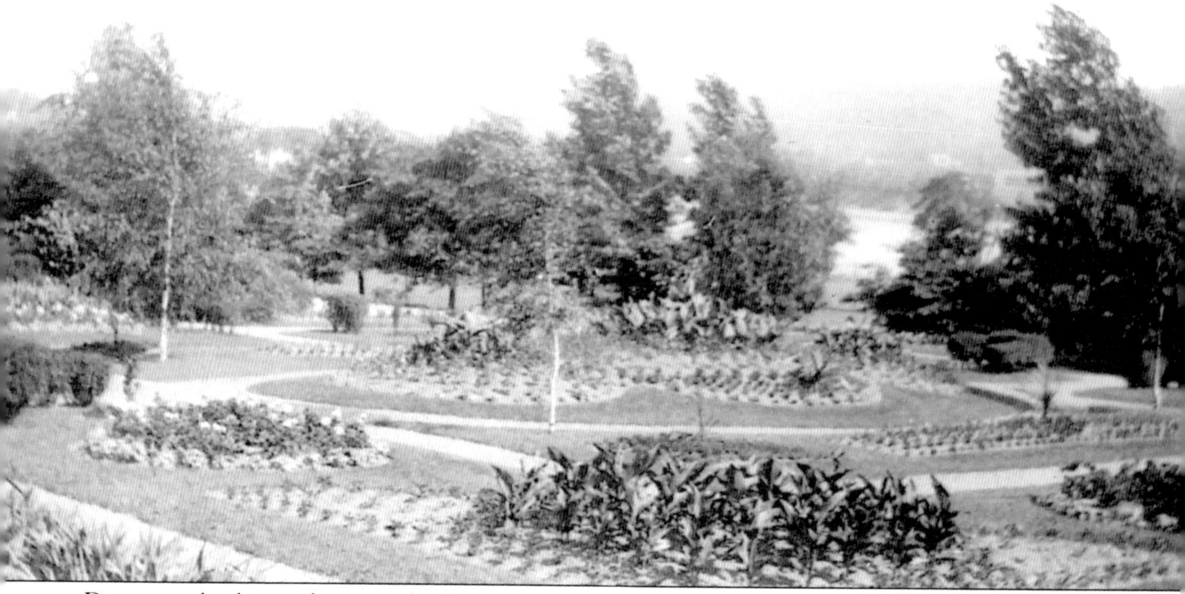

Dixmont also boasted immaculately groomed Victorian gardens. Shown here are the gardens in front of Reed Hall. In a letter later transcribed by Anita Reed Harder, J. A. Reed, son of Dr. Joseph Allison Reed, Dixmont's first superintendent, wrote that the gardens were comprised of "thousands of verbenas, geraniums, gladiolus, tuberoses, coleus, asters, petunias, phlox, pinks, acaranthus, Sweet Williams," and more. The importance of the flowers and landscaping at Dixmont was always a part of patient treatment, not just for aesthetic appeal. Many of the flowers on the property were grown in the greenhouse. "The money and labor spent in thus decorating and brightening the surroundings of the hospital brings a beautiful reward in the pleasure imparted to the patients who walk among the flowers, admiring and conversing about the lovely display so lavishly spread before them," Reed wrote. (Courtesy the Stroyne family collection.)

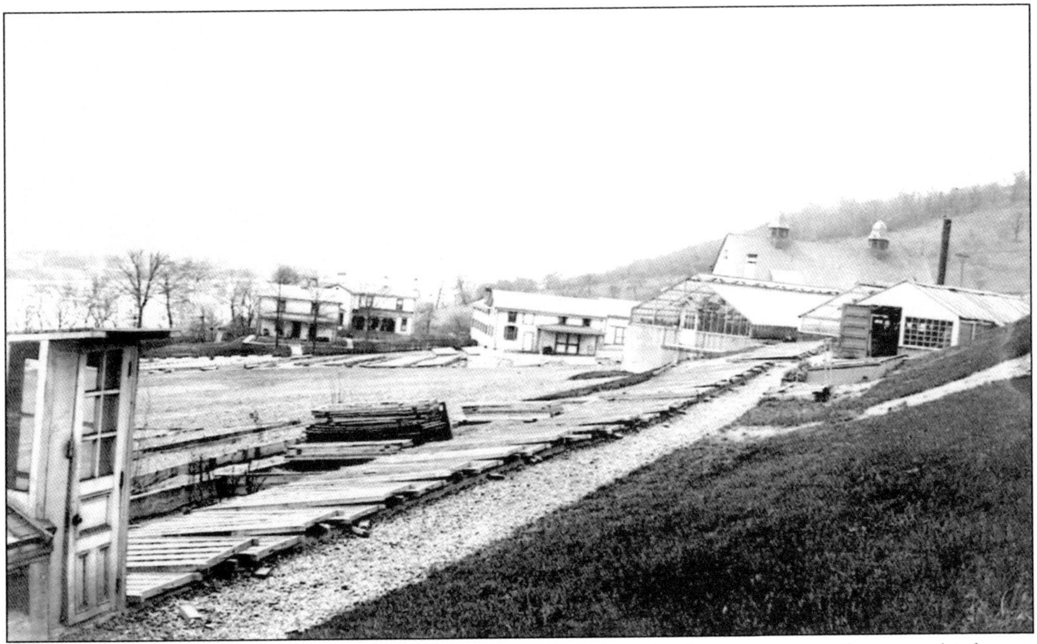

In addition to the flower gardens on the grounds, Dixmont had its own greenhouse, which was near the dairy barn. The greenhouse became such a staple of the hospital's operation, it was subject to a 2,484-square-foot addition in 1877. The addition allowed a greater portion of flowers to be grown over the winter season in preparation for the spring months. Flowers also were utilized on the wards as a means to beautify the patients' surroundings.

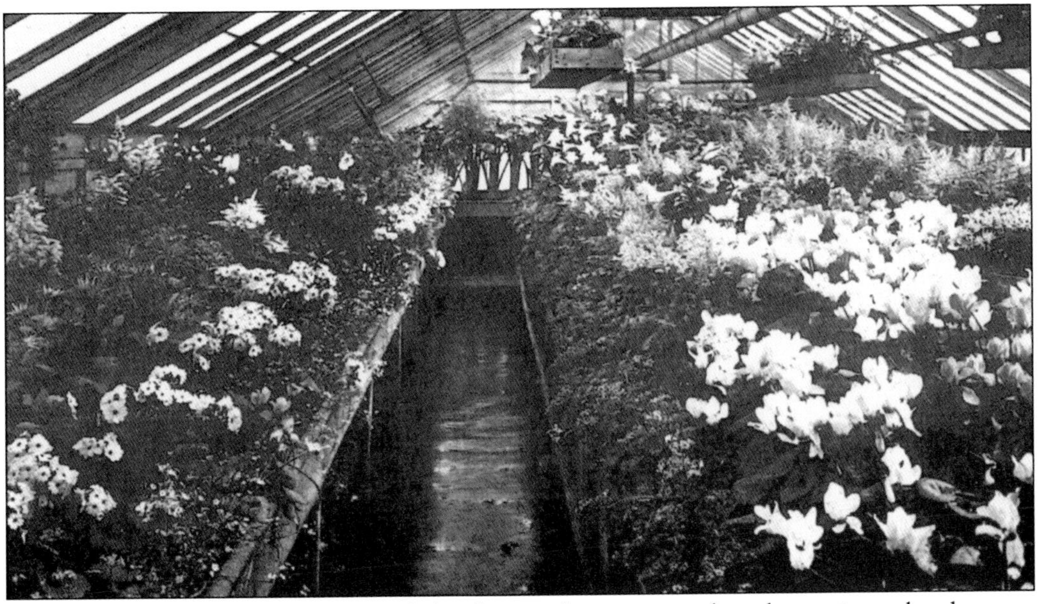

Inside the greenhouse grew many of the flowers that were used as decorations elsewhere on the property. The greenhouse was built in 1903 and primarily funded by Henry Phipps, known for Phipps Conservatory, one of America's oldest botanical gardens and greenhouses. Phipps grew up in poverty but became one of the region's many steel-wealthy philanthropists. The greenhouse stood until 1967, when it was demolished.

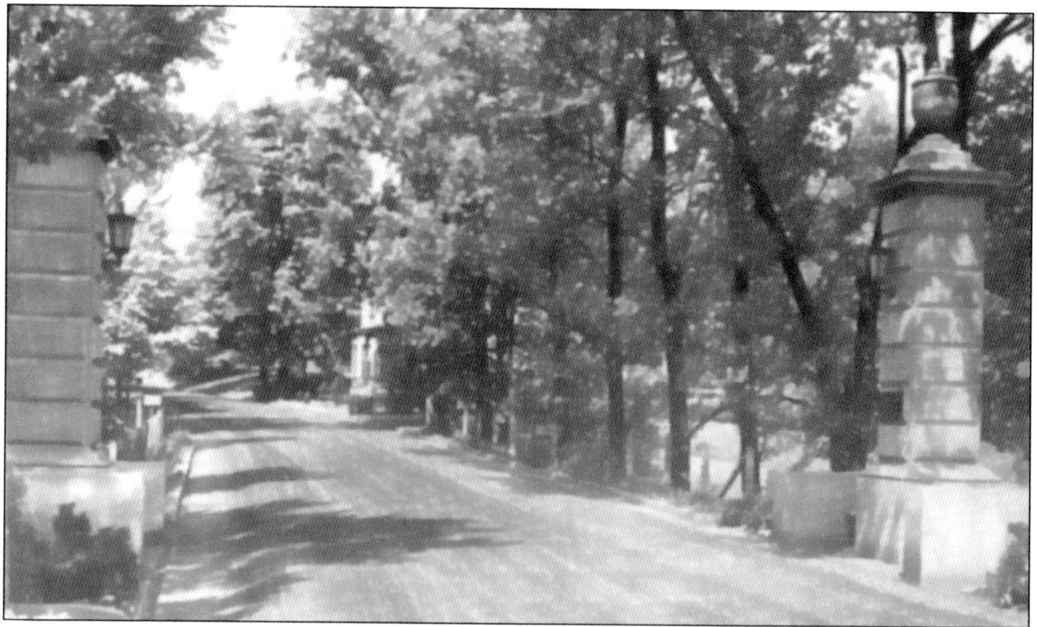

The main entrance to Dixmont was along what is now called Huntington Avenue in Emsworth Borough. The first sight visitors saw were two concrete columns topped with finial urns. This gateway was known as the Reed Memorial Gate. The superintendent's house, known as the Reed House, which later became known as the Rosenzweig House, is in the background to the right. It was named after Dr. Leonard Rosenzweig, who served as superintendent of Warren and Dixmont State Hospitals. He was a charter member of the Pittsburgh Psychiatric Society. Rosenzweig died in his home in Grand Rapids, Michigan, on May 18, 2001, at the age of 97.

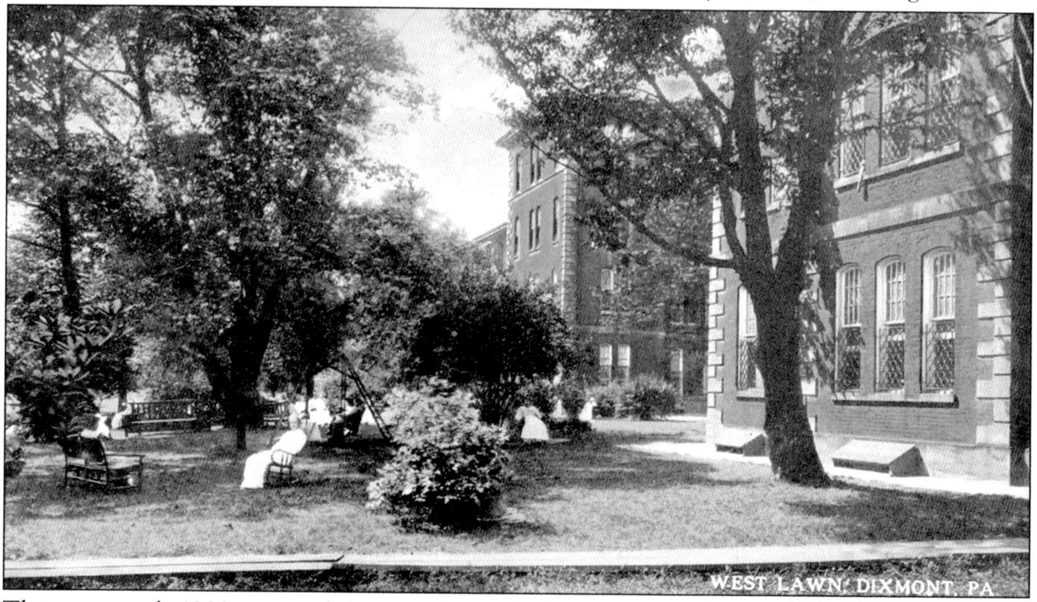

This is an early-1900s view of the west lawn of Dixmont with Reed Hall in the background. Nursing students can be seen sitting on the benches. A nurses' training school was first established at Dixmont in October 1895. The first graduates of the school, 3 men and 13 women, completed their training on May 7, 1897. The school was phased out in 1934.

This is another view of the West Lawn of Dixmont, with nurses dwarfed by the expansive landscaping on the site. Not only were flowers and shrubbery planted on the premises, fruit plants such as raspberries were planted on site for patients to harvest and eat berries. In 1878, more than 12,000 raspberry bushes were planted at Dixmont.

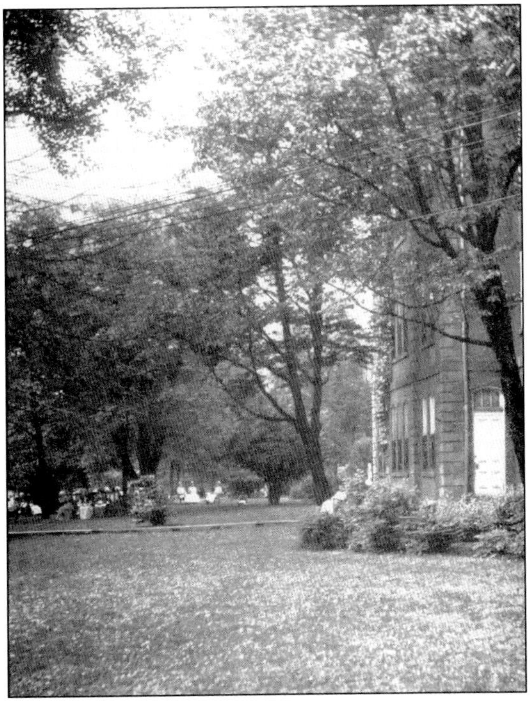

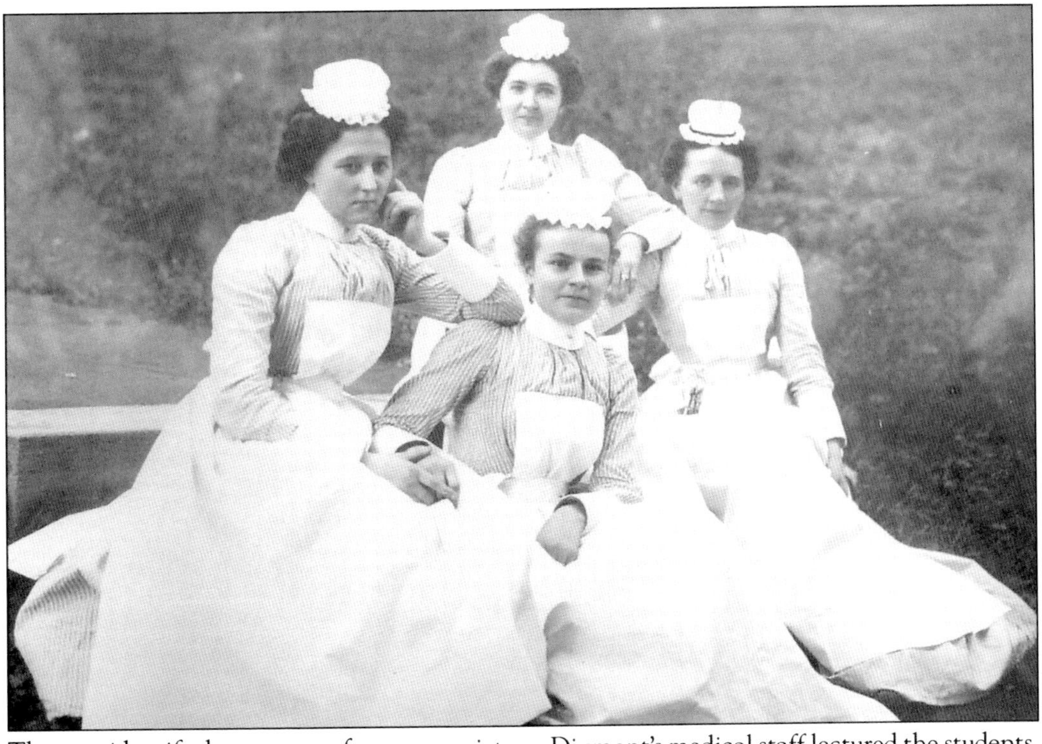

These unidentified nurses pose for a group picture. Dixmont's medical staff lectured the students. Other prominent medical figures lectured on an invitational basis. These doctors came from Pittsburgh and what was then known as Allegheny City, later annexed by Pittsburgh. Many of these doctors were invited by Dr. Henry Hutchinson, who also lectured at the school.

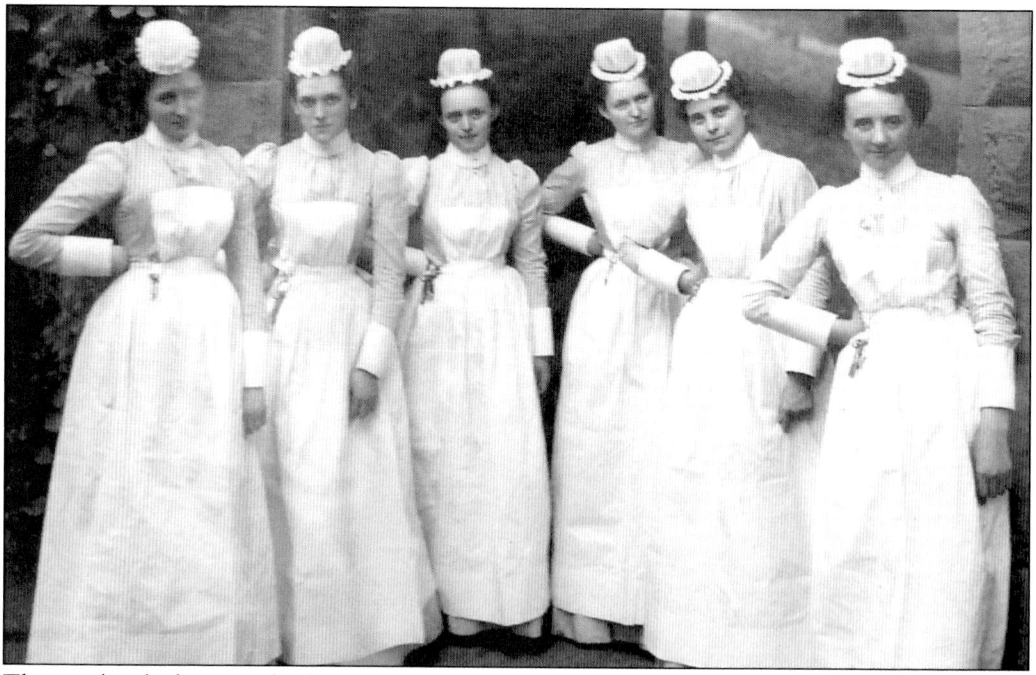

This undated photograph shows six Dixmont nurses. Not only did the nurses at Dixmont take care of the patients, they gave back to the institution to help see that it succeeded. In 1871, a library for the female wards was created by Dorothea Lynde Dix and Mary Moorhead. Dixmont nurses collected $8 to be used on books for the library. That money would equal $130 in today's value. Given the fact that nurses' salaries were very little at the time, $8 was no small contribution.

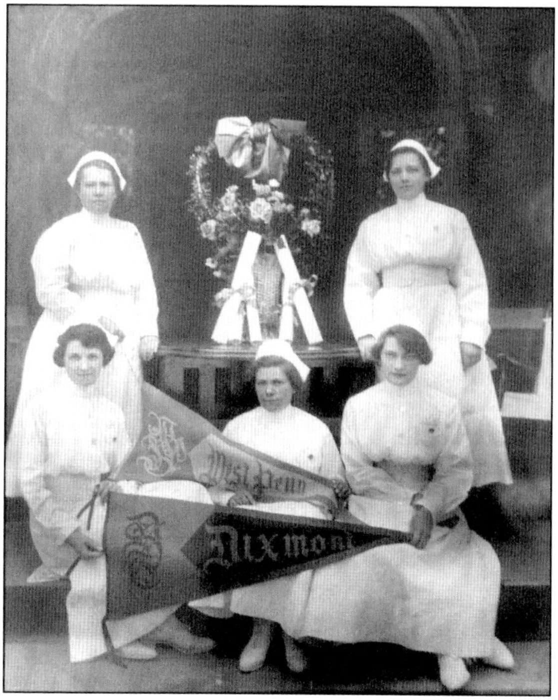

These five nursing graduates pose with their dual alma matter pennants: one for the Western Pennsylvania Hospital and one for Dixmont State Hospital. The picture is undated, and the nurses are unidentified.

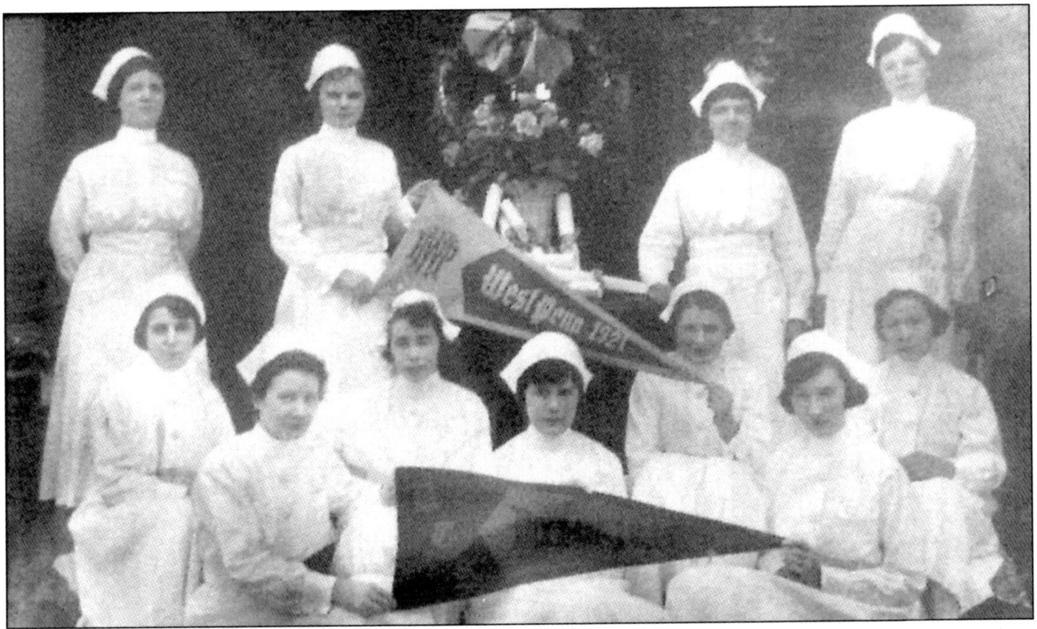

This was the female nursing class of 1921. While unidentified on the photograph, the class included Edna Katherine Durst, Ethel Elizabeth Gibb, Ruth E. Pickering, Bessie Bell Pickering, Mabel B. Davis, Elizabeth A. Smith, Elizabeth M. Nicholson, Gertrude L. Davis, Matreda B. Beckman, Mabel Amelia Bock, and Ella Luzurah Hite. Students came from Pennsylvania, West Virginia, Ohio, and Maryland.

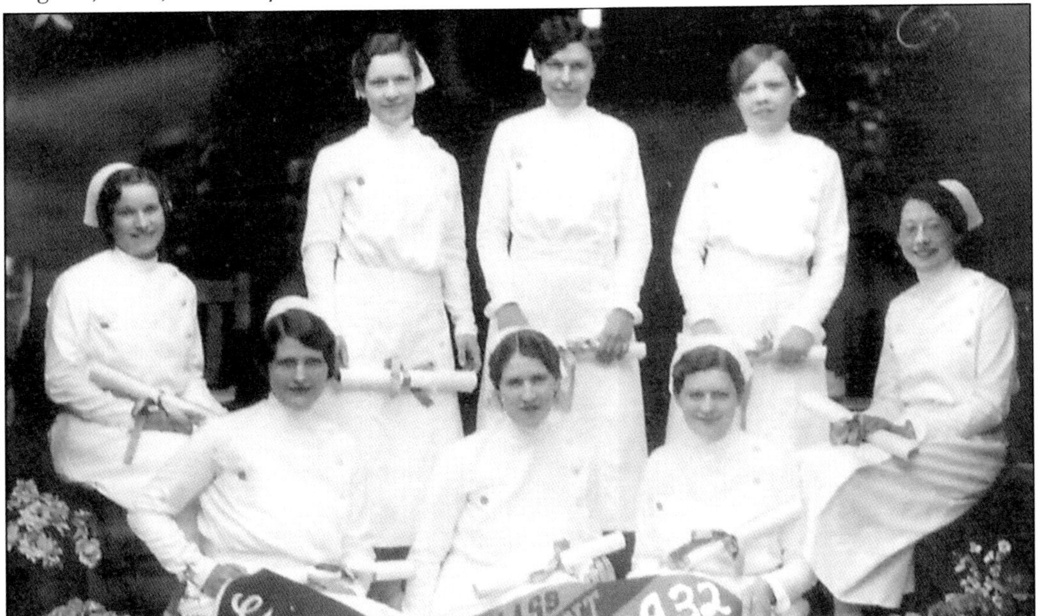

Pictured here is the female nursing class of 1932. They are unidentified on the photograph, but records show that the class consisted of Edwyna Alberta Alexander, Winifred Ceceila Barker, Eleanor Elizabeth Egolf, Sophia Theresa Froncek, Emma Florella Griffin, Mabel Josephine McCullough, and Pearl Marilda McBride. All were from Pennsylvania. The last class to go through Dixmont, the class of 1934, only had three students.

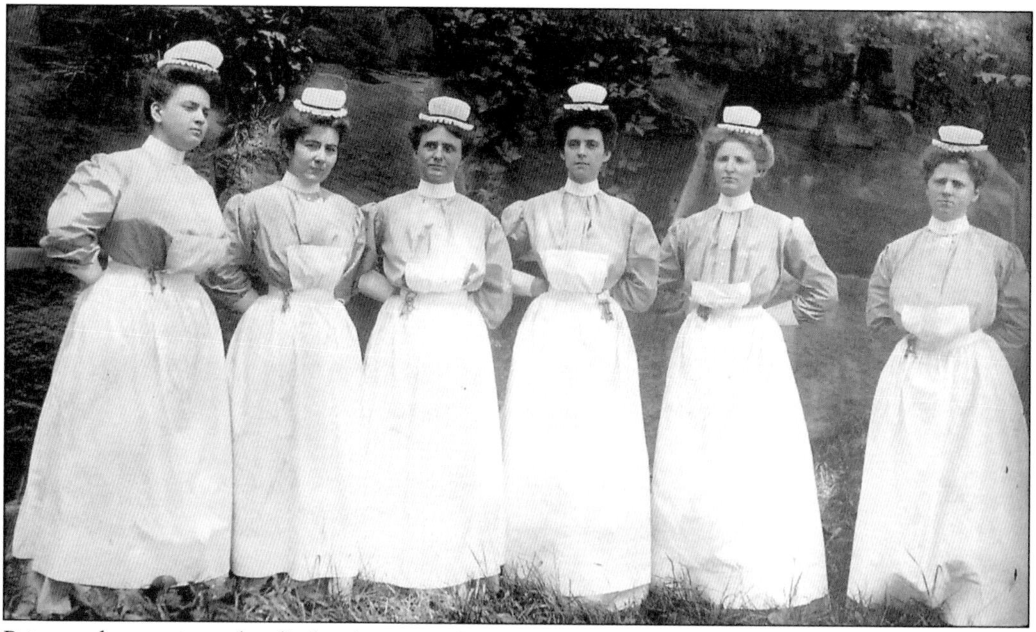

Prior to the nursing school's development, Dixmont officials instituted a lecture course designed to train nurses in the proper care of the insane. Developed in 1887, this course was key to the proper and dignified treatment of patients. Pictured here are six unidentified nurses.

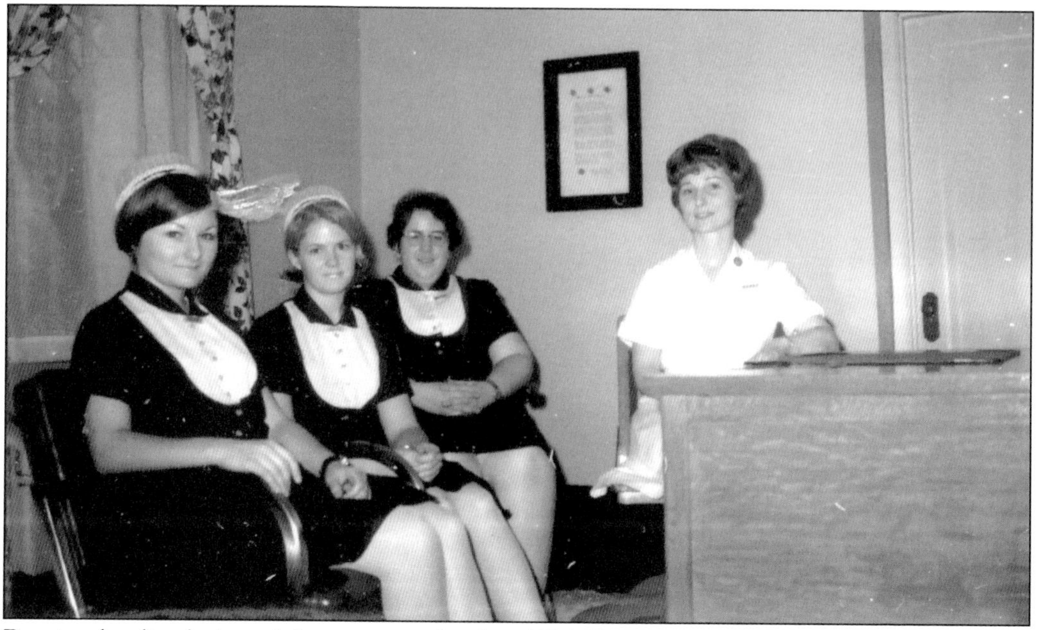

Despite the dissolution of the nursing school in 1934, Dixmont remained an important part of nursing education until its doors closed in 1984. These three students are from Pennsylvania State University and are working on their psychology affiliation training at Dixmont in February 1968. From left to right are Faye Baldwin, Hannah Kilgore, Judith Pfeil, and ? Millot, their instructor. (Courtesy Helen Wolf.)

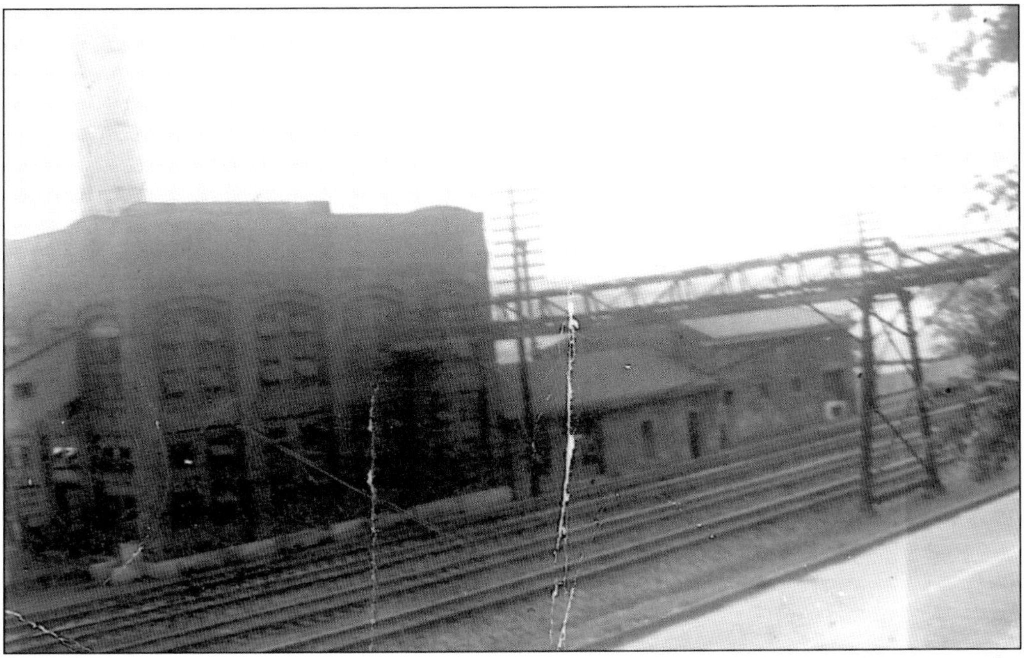

Pictured here is the old Dixmont power plant, which was situated along the Ohio River. The building, which was constructed in 1917, was abandoned in 1953. Like most of Dixmont's buildings, the building became a target for vandalism. On January 24, 1966, the western section of the roof caught fire and caused major damage to the building. The power plant was eventually demolished.

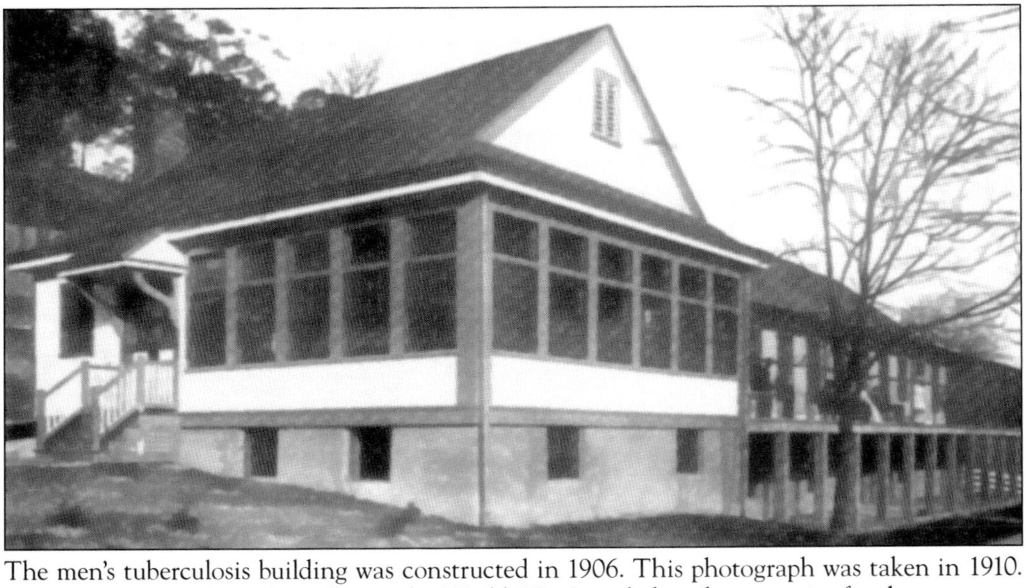

The men's tuberculosis building was constructed in 1906. This photograph was taken in 1910. The outbreak of tuberculosis during the World War I era led to the necessity for the structure. It housed about 30 patients and three staff members. Dixmont was not immune from pandemics and took them very seriously. Prior to the tuberculosis outbreaks, small pox threatened the country in 1871. Dixmont had not one case of small pox and credits the prompt vaccination of patients with its success. Dr. J. C. Hupp of Wheeling, West Virginia, was publicly lauded for supplying vaccine for more than 500 patients and several hundred employees.

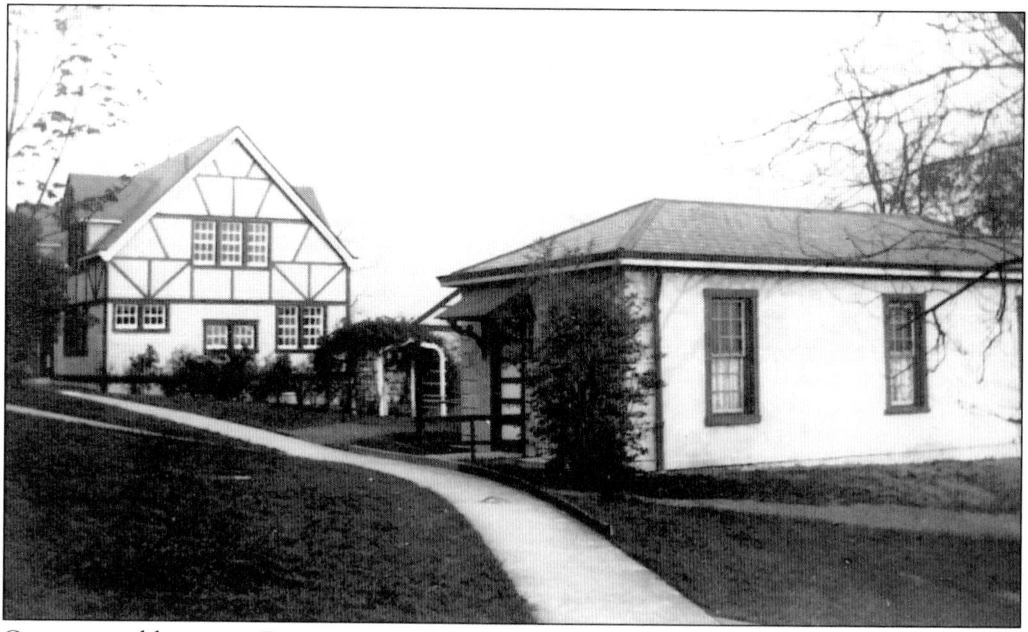

Cottages and houses at Dixmont were reused for programs such as the Hospital Improvement Program, or HIP, which utilized colored tokens and reinforced positive patient behavior by allowing them to purchase daily necessities and some luxuries with the tokens they earned. The program was implemented in the late 1960s. The tuberculosis buildings were eventually converted into geriatric buildings.

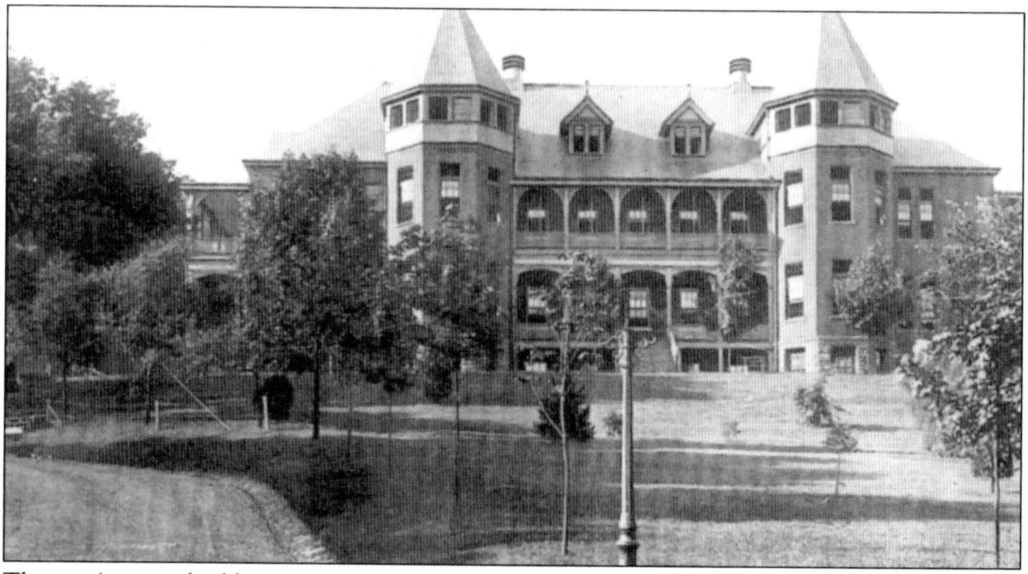

The men's annex building was a wooden structure that measured 41 feet by 125 feet by 50 feet and was built in 1889. After two years of abandonment, the building was scavenged for salvageable material and was demolished two years after it was shut down at a cost of $15,000. The building was considered a fire hazard.

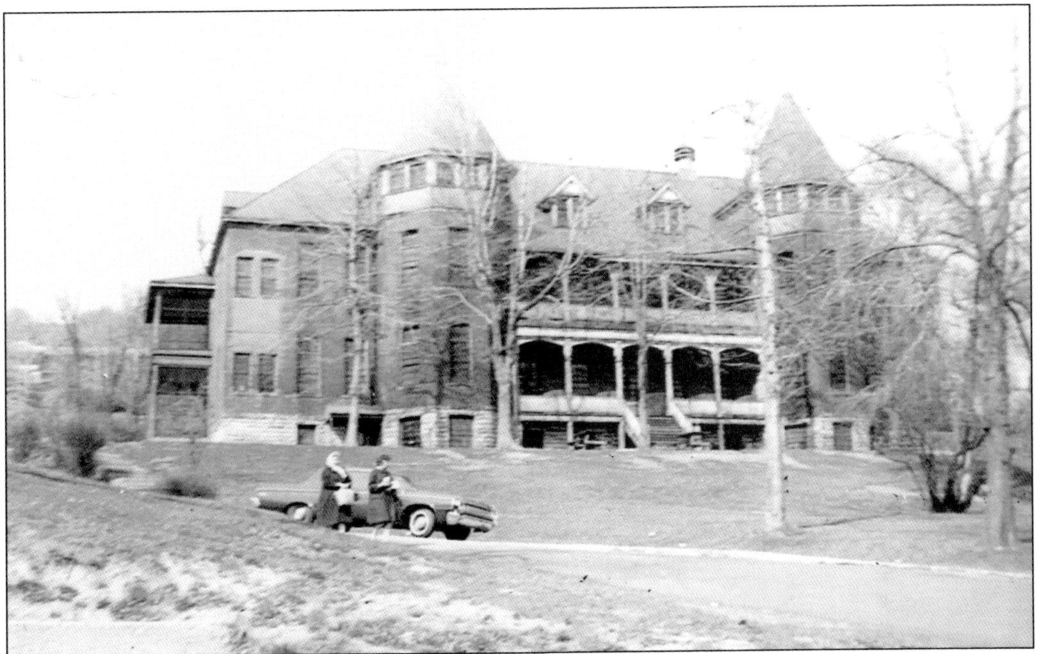

In 1949, the men's annex received a considerable upgrade through funding provided by the Pennsylvania Department of Property and Supplies. The cost of the remodel was $84,249 and included bath and toilet replacements and two new brick-enclosed fire escapes with a steel fire door on each of the building's three floors.

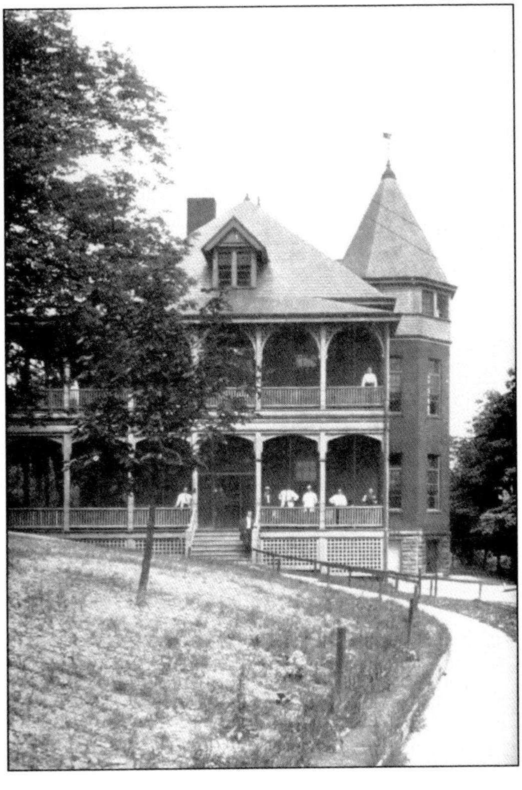

The men's annex also housed its own kitchen and staff quarters. Like most of Dixmont's buildings, over time, the annex became too costly to operate and was abandoned.

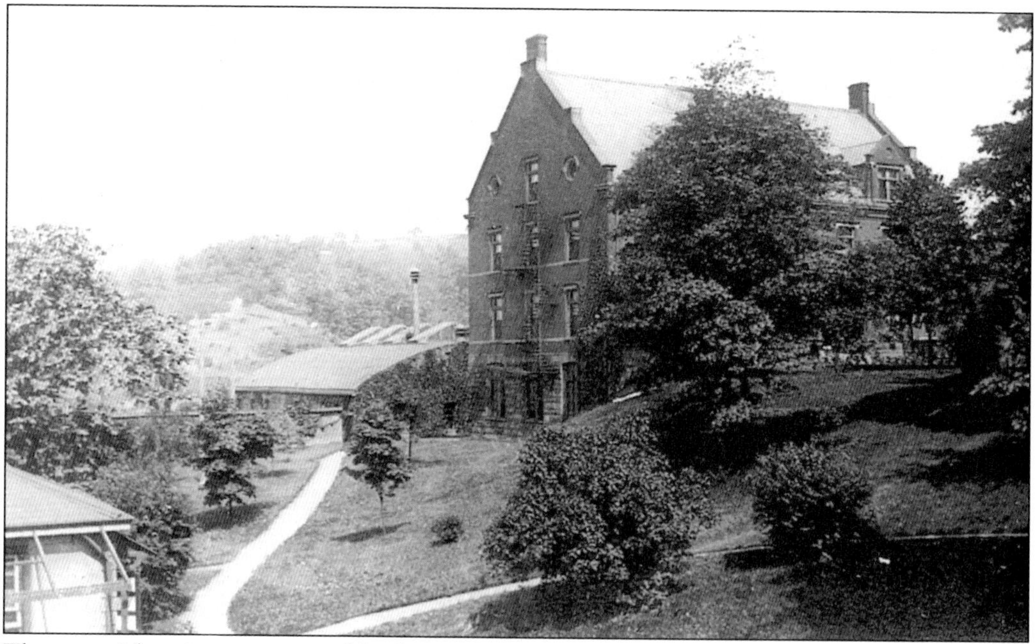

The nurses' dormitory was one of the longest-surviving buildings on the property and, eventually, was renovated and creatively reused as the Dixieland Canteen, a small general store where ice cream, hot dogs, and other various items could be purchased for little expense. In May 1983, the building was surveyed for the Pennsylvania Office of Historic Preservation, where it was described as "curiously attractive." It was demolished between July 11 and September 16, 1983, at a cost of $10,900.

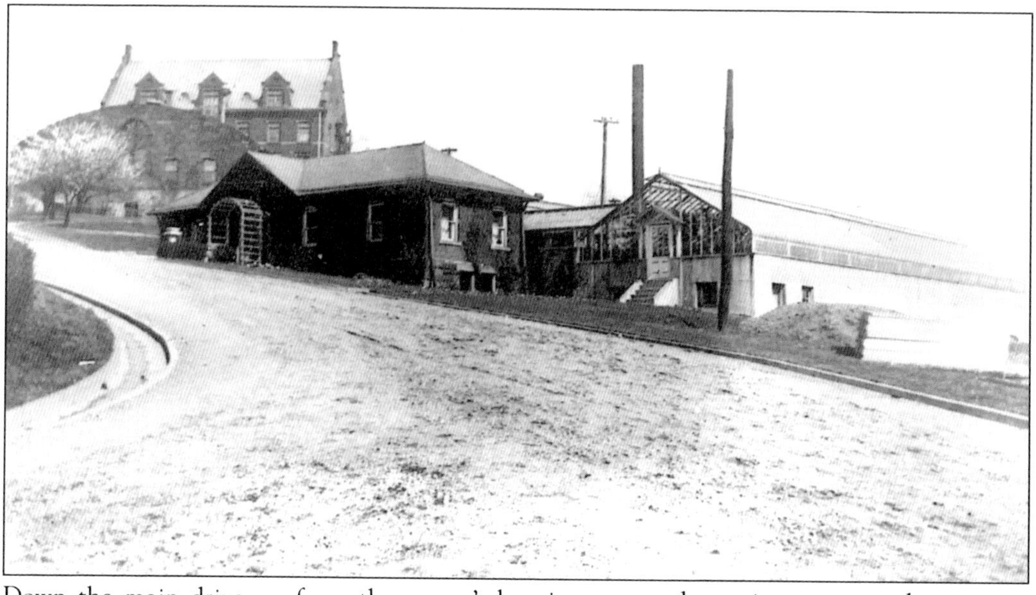

Down the main driveway from the nurses' dormitory were the maintenance and carpentry shop and greenhouse. According to a June 1983 historic survey, the building's original use was as Dixmont's original laundry building. The maintenance and carpenter shop were originally constructed in 1878. These buildings were ineligible for inclusion on the National Register of Historic Places.

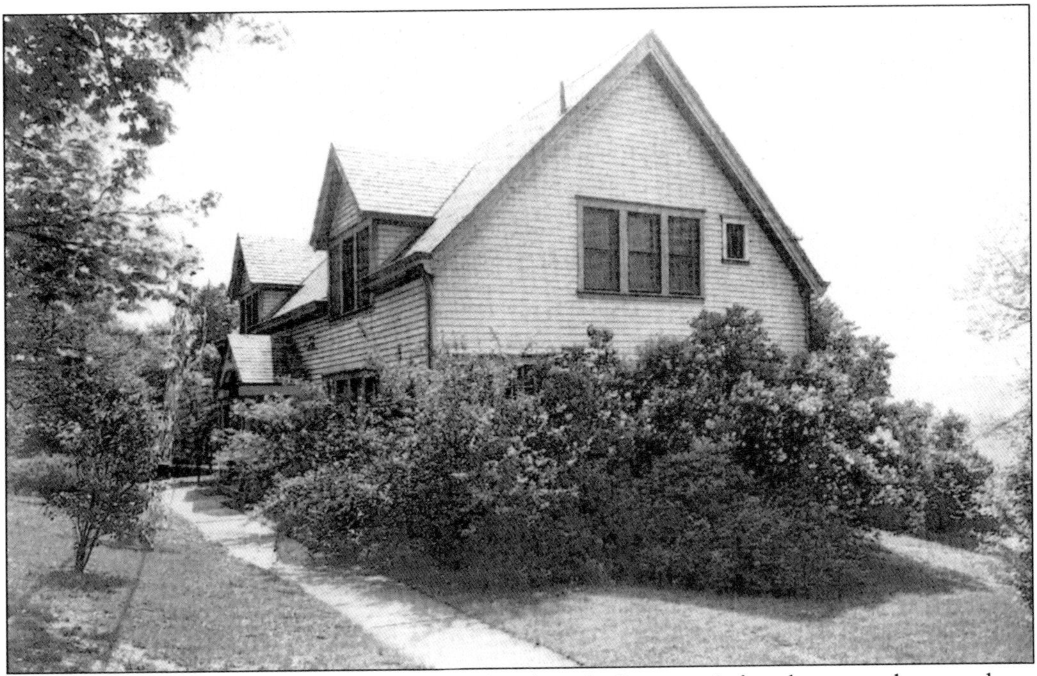

The occupational house for women provided a place for Dixmont's females to produce products while recuperating. "This form of employment adds so much to their general health and in making their lives endurable," superintendent Henry Hutchinson wrote in a 1932 report. The two-and-one-half-story frame building was demolished in 1967.

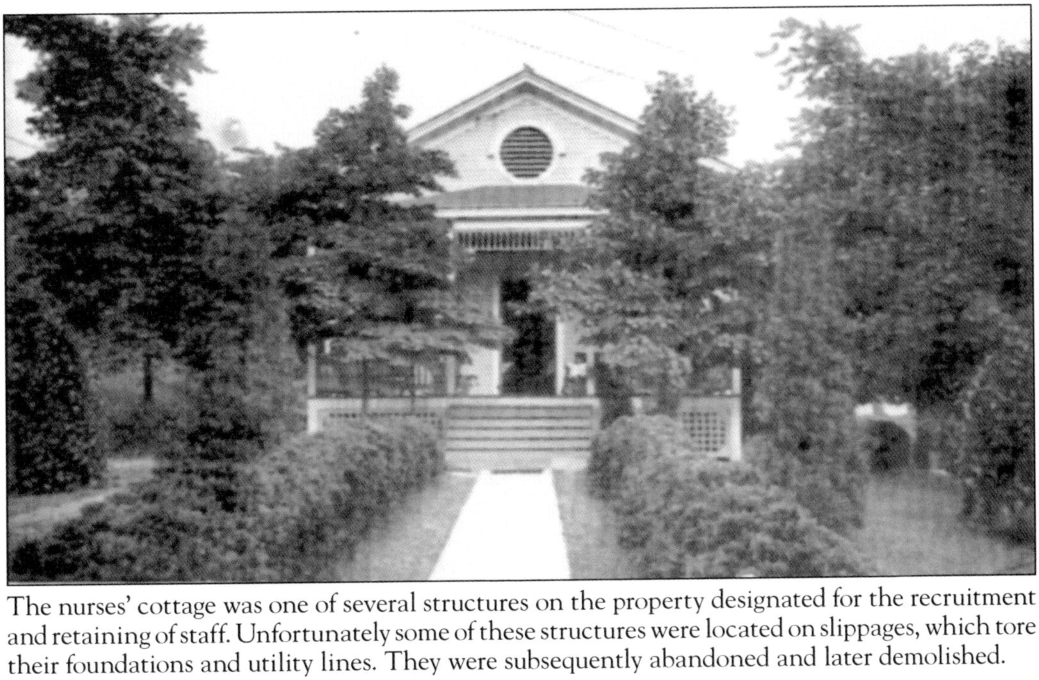

The nurses' cottage was one of several structures on the property designated for the recruitment and retaining of staff. Unfortunately some of these structures were located on slippages, which tore their foundations and utility lines. They were subsequently abandoned and later demolished.

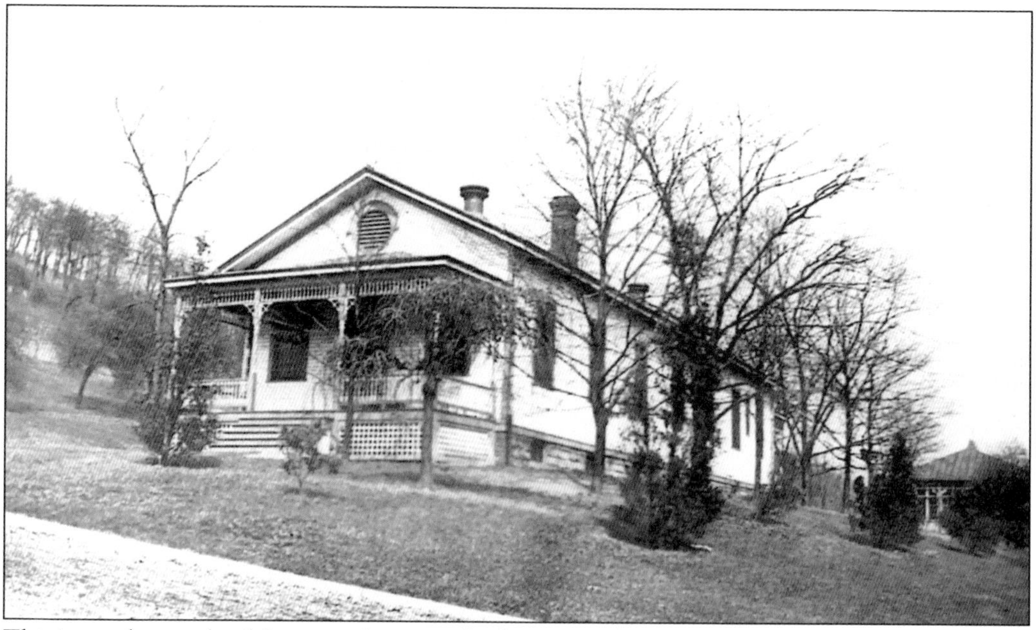

This is another angle of the nurses' cottage. In the 1940s, the administration explored purchasing houses off-campus to offer housing to senior psychiatric professionals. These houses were located on Ohio River Boulevard. The cottages were reused over time for programs such as the Hospital Improvement Program.

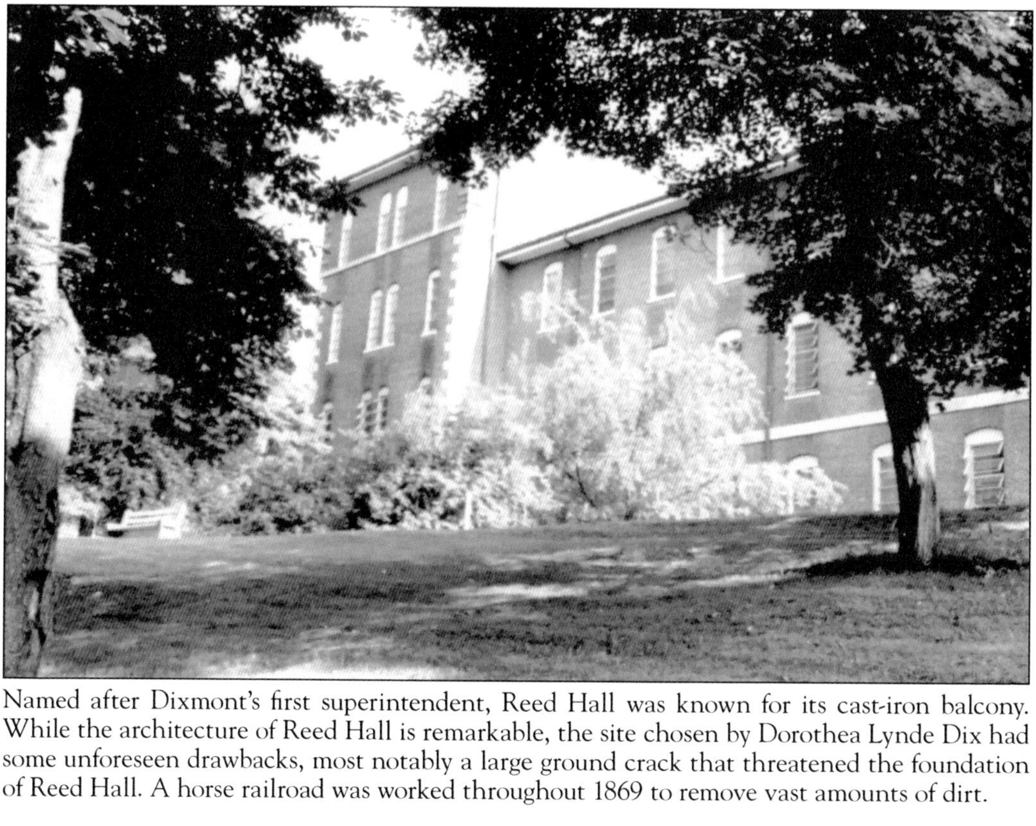

Named after Dixmont's first superintendent, Reed Hall was known for its cast-iron balcony. While the architecture of Reed Hall is remarkable, the site chosen by Dorothea Lynde Dix had some unforeseen drawbacks, most notably a large ground crack that threatened the foundation of Reed Hall. A horse railroad was worked throughout 1869 to remove vast amounts of dirt.

The Riverhouse was a little-photographed structure that served as a patient residence. According to former Dixmont employees, the Riverhouse was a patient's last step on the road to release. Eventually the Riverhouse was razed. Part of Dixmont's property included several residential-type homes and cottages. Some, like the Riverhouse, were used as alternate housing for patients. Others were used to house doctors and their families. (Courtesy Helen Wolf.)

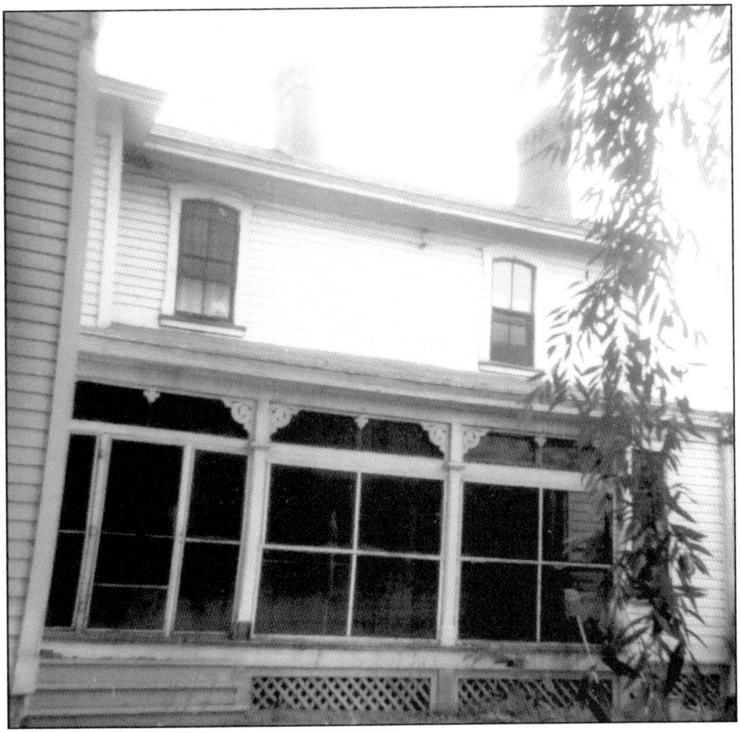

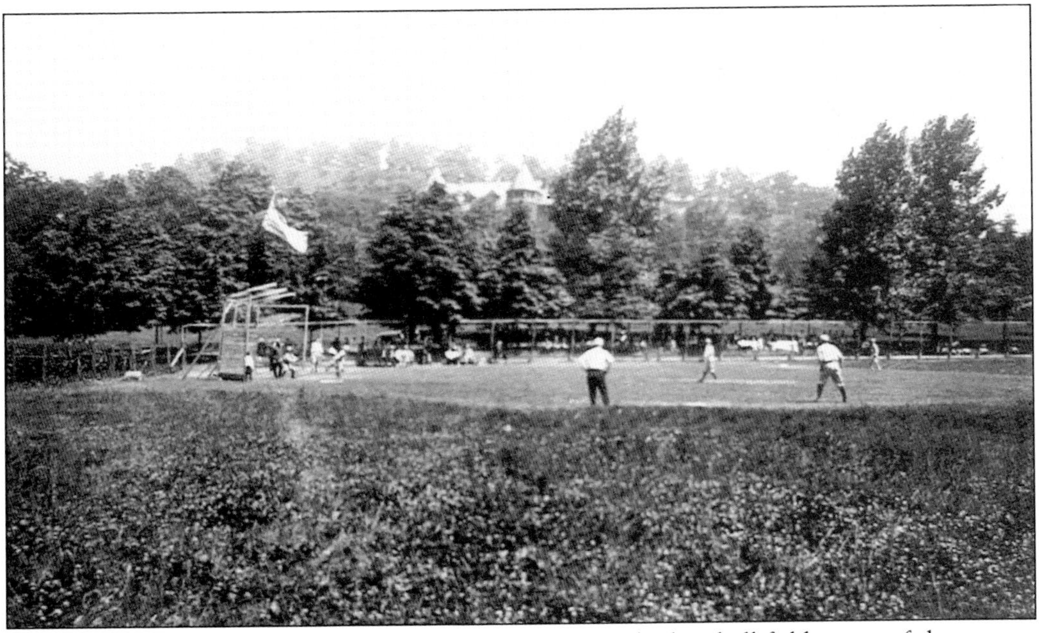

The great American pastime was not lost on Dixmont. The baseball field is one of the aspects of the property that came full circle during the hospital's history. Once part of the hospital property, the ball field was let go and became the future site of the Hutchinson Building. Years after Dixmont's closing, a portion of the abandoned Dixmont property was sold to Emsworth Borough to make way for Mayernik Field, a baseball field situated at the end of Huntington Avenue. The field is directly adjacent to where the Hutchinson Building used to stand.

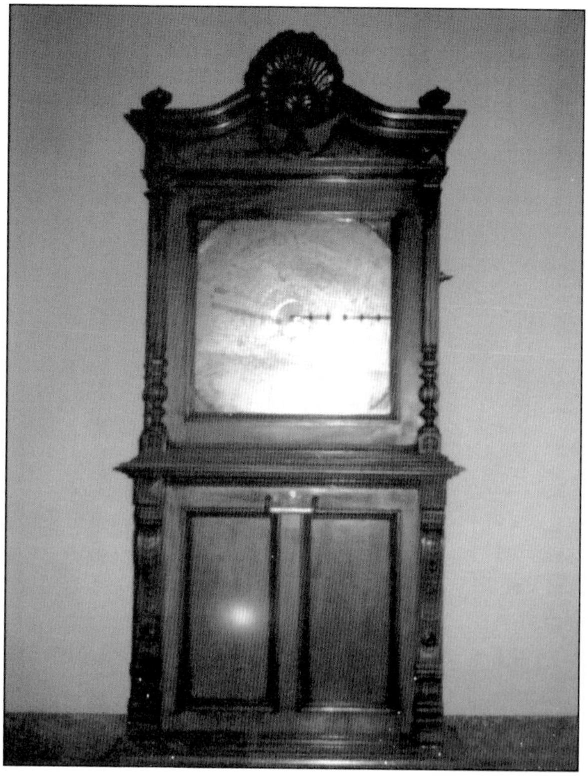

This photograph shows the upright music player that was left over from Dixmont's early history. Music was an integral part of Dixmont's therapeutic environment. Dixmont's wards had pianos, guitars, and violins, as well as other items of entertainment, such as pool tables and magic lantern shows. Dr. Henry Hutchinson continued to carry out a regime of activities engineered by Dr. Joseph Allison Reed before his death. (Courtesy Helen Wolf.)

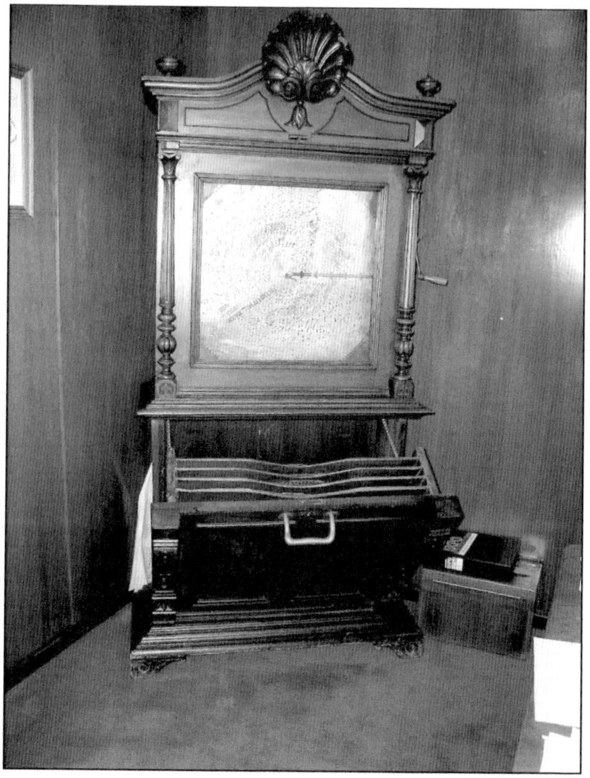

Today the upright music player stands in a wood-paneled corner of the office of the executive director of Mayview State Hospital. The player is made of mahogany and plays 27-inch disks of music. The disks are made of metal and are perforated. The entire machine operates in much the same fashion as a small windup music box. Today versions of these items that are in excellent condition can sell for as high as $25,000.

This detail of the upright music disk shows John Philip Sousa's "Liberty Bell March." No one knows the last time the disk was changed or the last time the march was played. What is known is that there is a collection of more than a dozen such disks, each with a diameter approaching three feet, cached within the bottom portion of the music player.

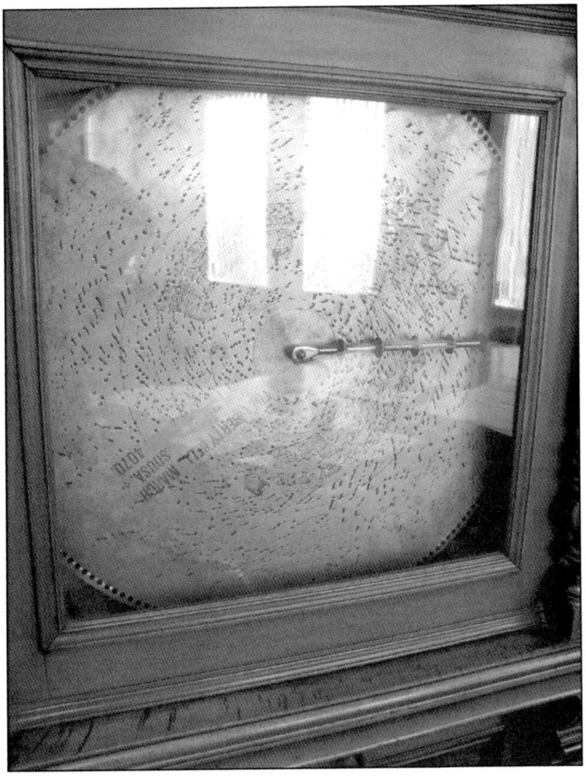

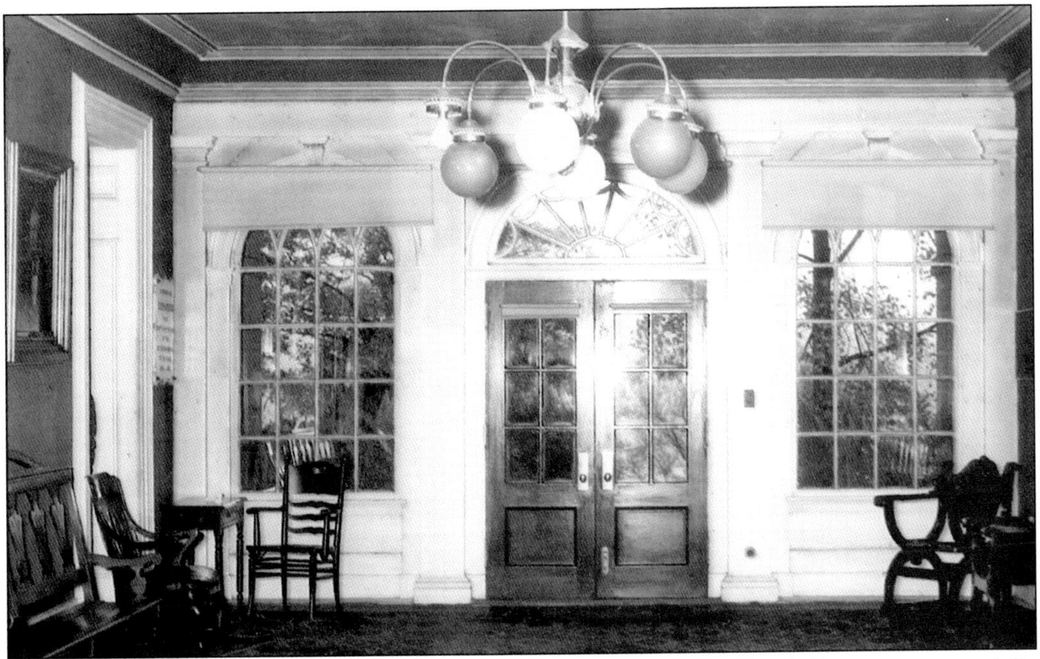

This interior of Reed Hall shows some of the exquisite furniture and style Dixmont enjoyed. In 1876, Dorothea Lynde Dix spent six weeks living here, supervising the hospital that bore her name. She died shortly thereafter in Trenton, New Jersey, but not before writing that Dixmont was a "noble charity" that embraced "the best good of the patient residents."

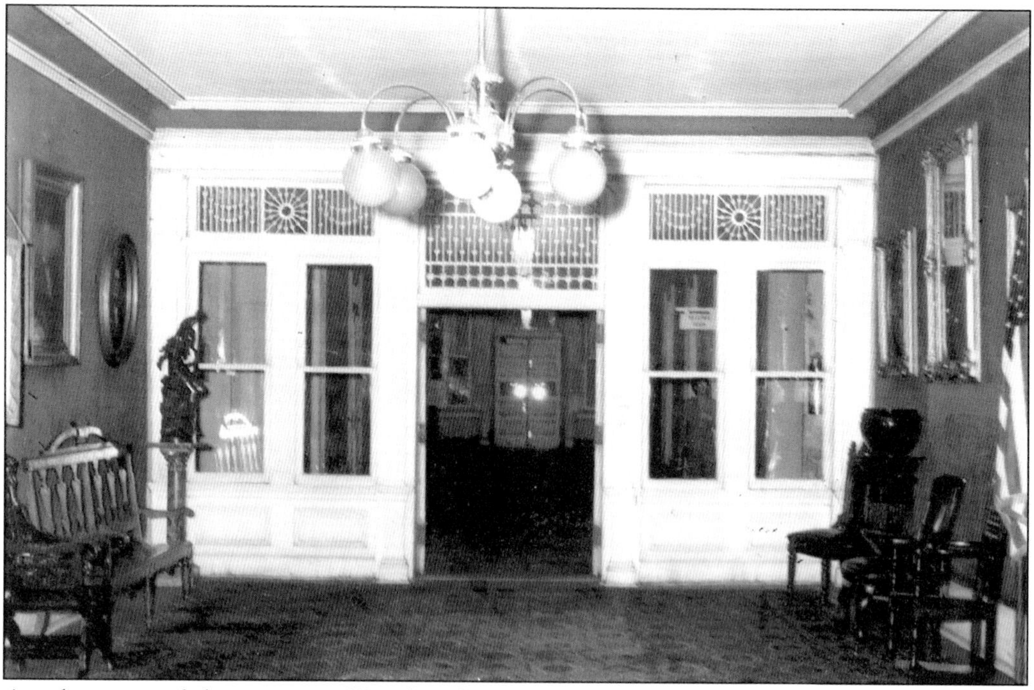

Another view of the interior of Reed Hall shows more of the furniture and several portraits hanging along the corridor. It was this dignity and decorum that Dr. Robert Weimer sought to recapture through his Renaissance Program. His efforts were so revered that Dr. Anibal Herrera wrote in a 1970 newsletter, "Surely [Dorothea Lynde Dix] will bless those who are continuing her work of love and care to the insane in the hospital that she established."

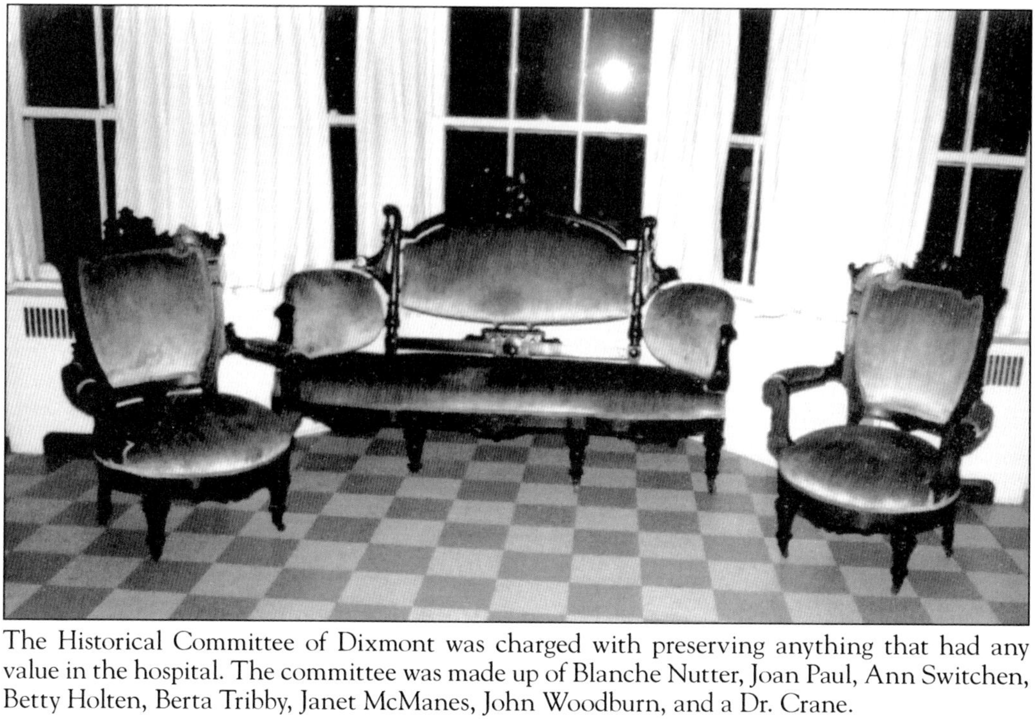

The Historical Committee of Dixmont was charged with preserving anything that had any value in the hospital. The committee was made up of Blanche Nutter, Joan Paul, Ann Switchen, Betty Holten, Berta Tribby, Janet McManes, John Woodburn, and a Dr. Crane.

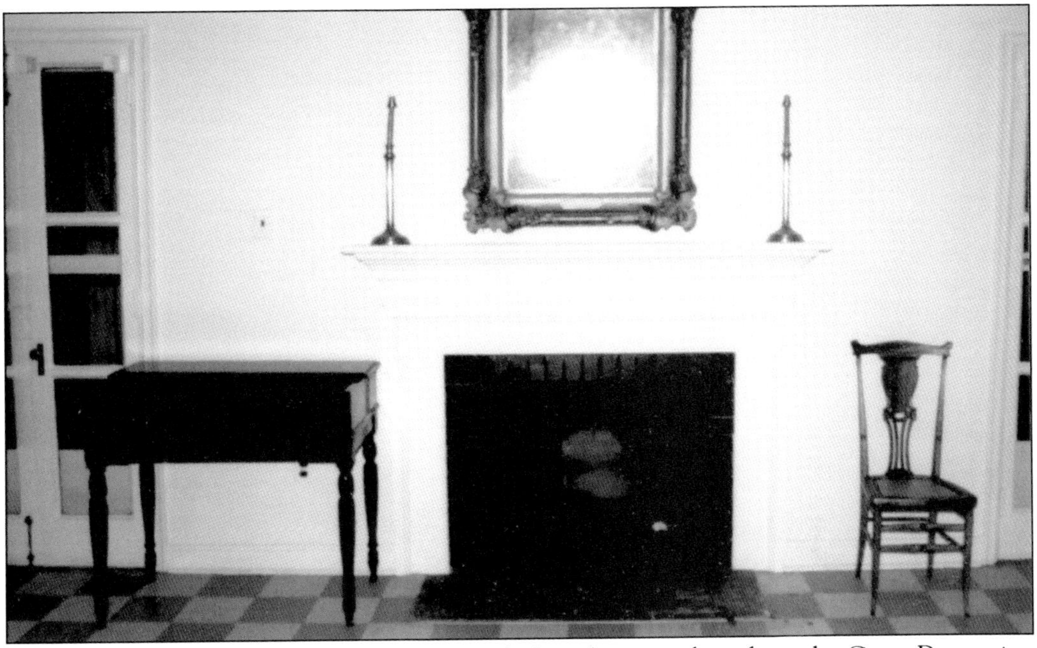

In 1934, David Reed, president of the hospital's board, wrote about how the Great Depression had begun to take its toll on Dixmont's finances. However, "the institution at this time is well furnished and most comfortable." Despite highs and lows in funding and circumstance, aesthetics remained a priority at Dixmont. High quality amenities such as furniture, recreational equipment, and the like were provided to the patients.

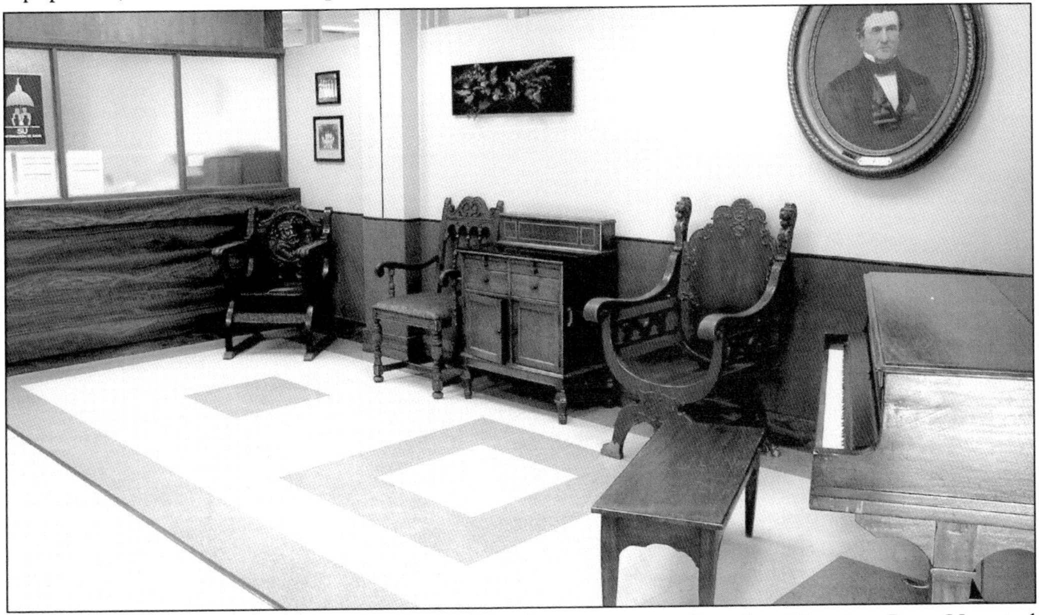

So much of Dixmont's antique furniture and artifacts were transferred to Mayview State Hospital that many pieces are located in heavily traveled areas of the hospital. Here a portrait of William Herron, furniture, and a piano sit in an alcove inside the Bengs Building at Mayview State Hospital. The former location of Herron's portrait was in the entrance of Reed Hall, along with the other members of the Dixmont executive committee and board of managers.

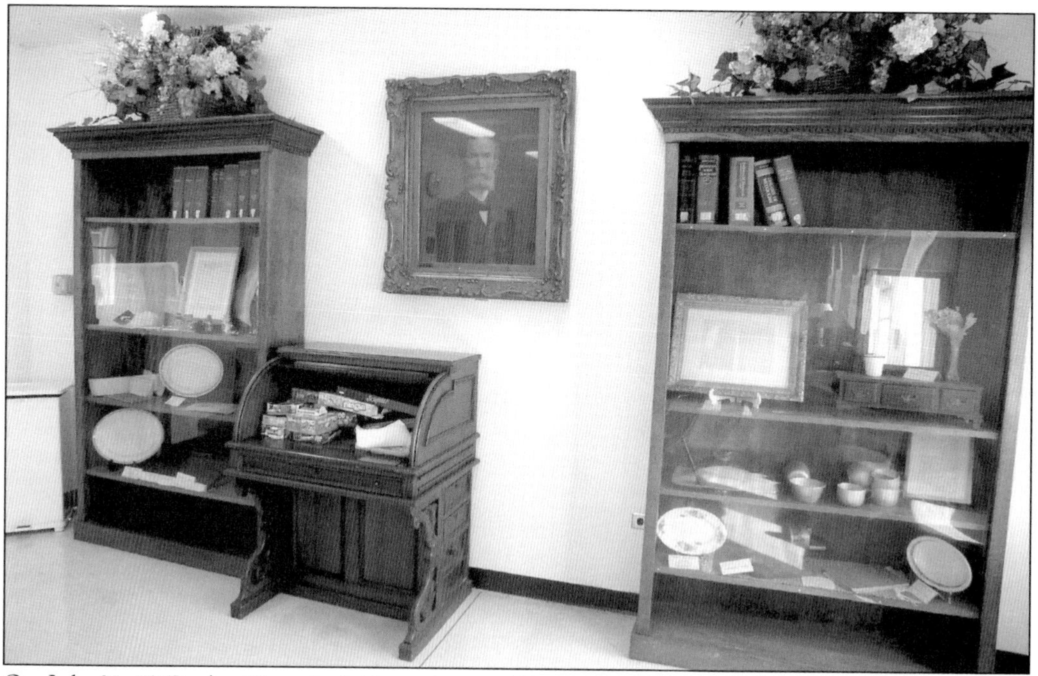

On July 21, 1967, the Historical Committee of Dixmont was founded. Prior to that, anything at Dixmont with historical value was treated haphazardly. "There are no records of the sale of items which could be termed either valuable or of historical interest," wrote librarian Ann Switchen in the August 1967 staff newsletter. "Because of lack of storage space, it has been the practice to destroy rather than retain."

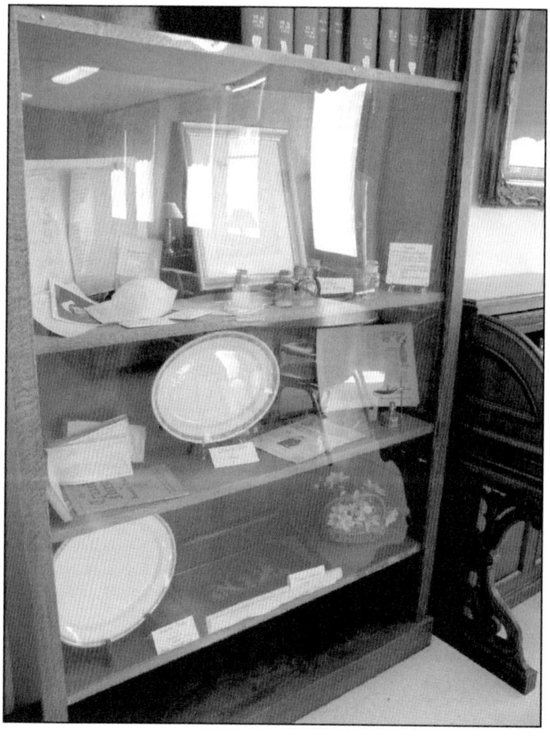

To protect its contents, the fronts of the bookcases were sealed with an acrylic panel. Inside are china platters, various notes, receipts, dinnerware, articles of agreement, and other miscellaneous items from Dixmont's past. All of the items in Mayview's Dixmont collection are cataloged and numbered.

While the top of this rolltop desk has been fixed permanently open, it is still used by hospital staff and patients. Perhaps once used by Dr. Joseph Allison Reed to draft a note or letter, it now stores puzzles and games such as checkers and Scrabble for patients to play.

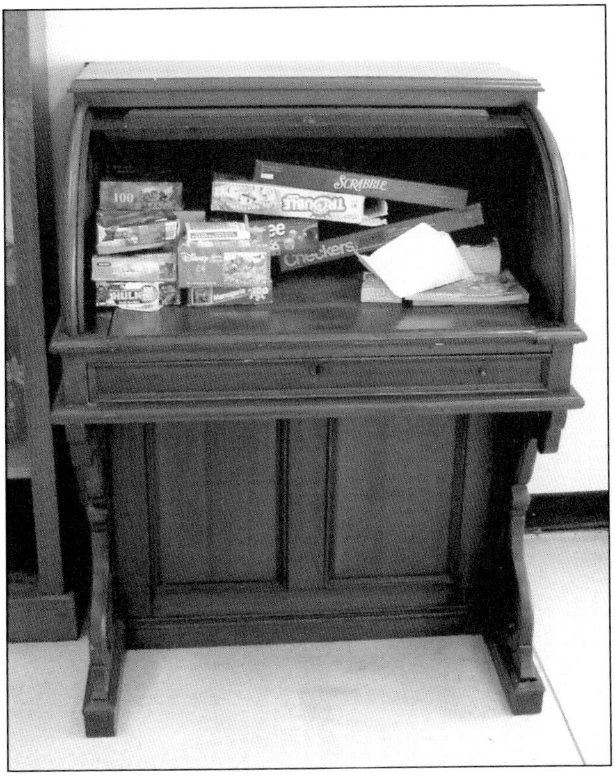

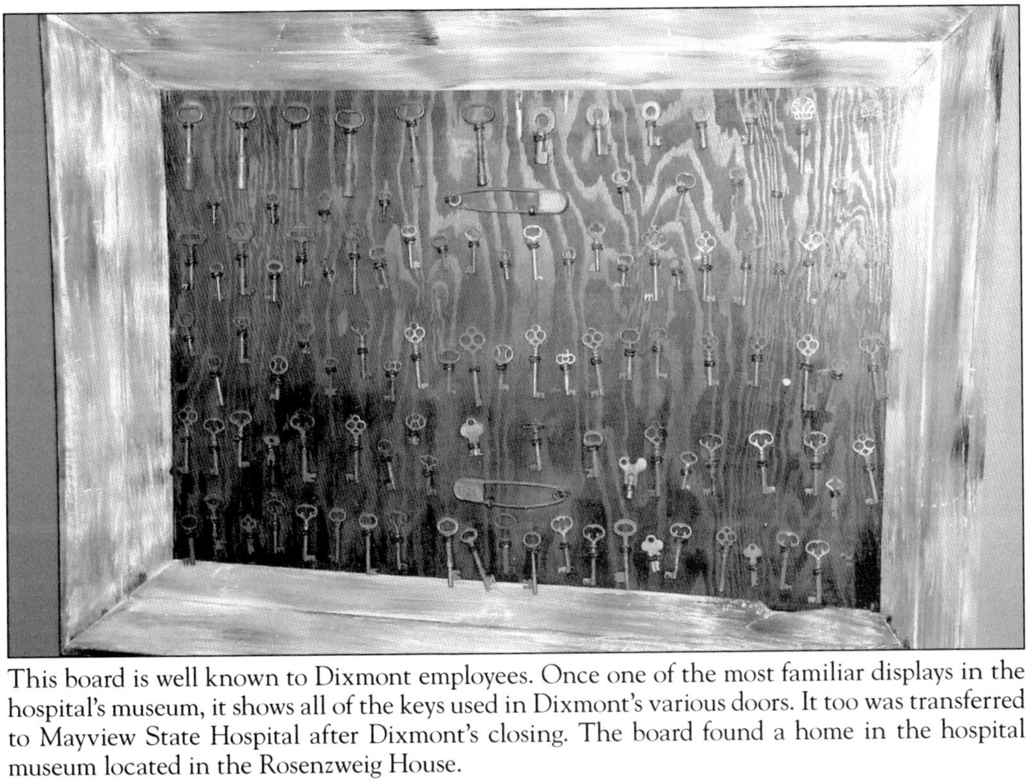

This board is well known to Dixmont employees. Once one of the most familiar displays in the hospital's museum, it shows all of the keys used in Dixmont's various doors. It too was transferred to Mayview State Hospital after Dixmont's closing. The board found a home in the hospital museum located in the Rosenzweig House.

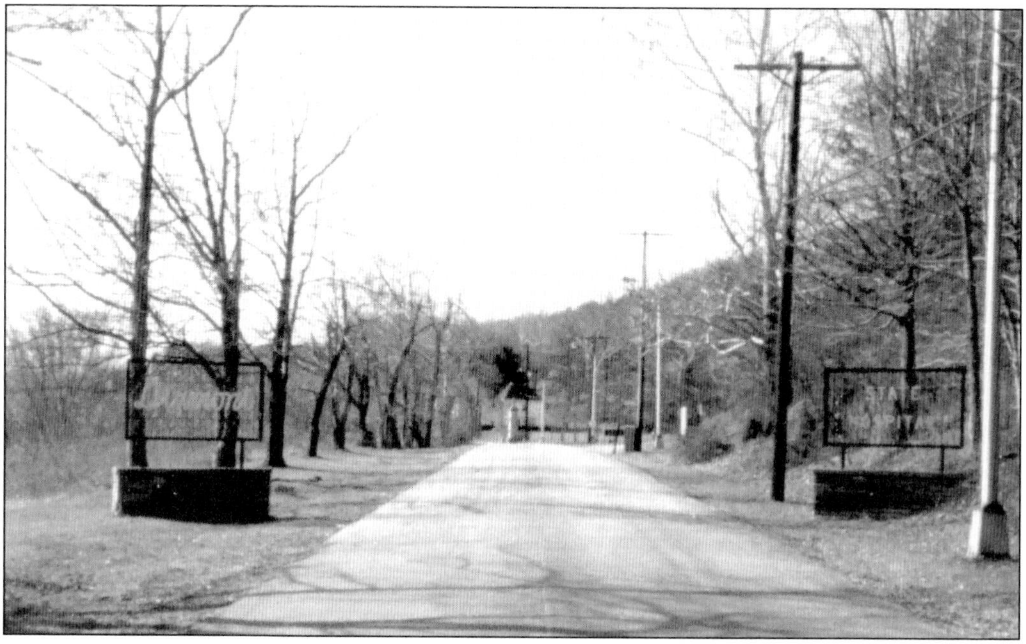

Huntington Avenue was not the main entrance to the hospital, but rather a visitor's entrance. However, delivery trucks found it a convenient route into the Dixmont campus, which irked neighbors. The solicitor for the Borough of Emsworth was urged to write the superintendent regarding the matter. (Courtesy Tracy Ferguson.)

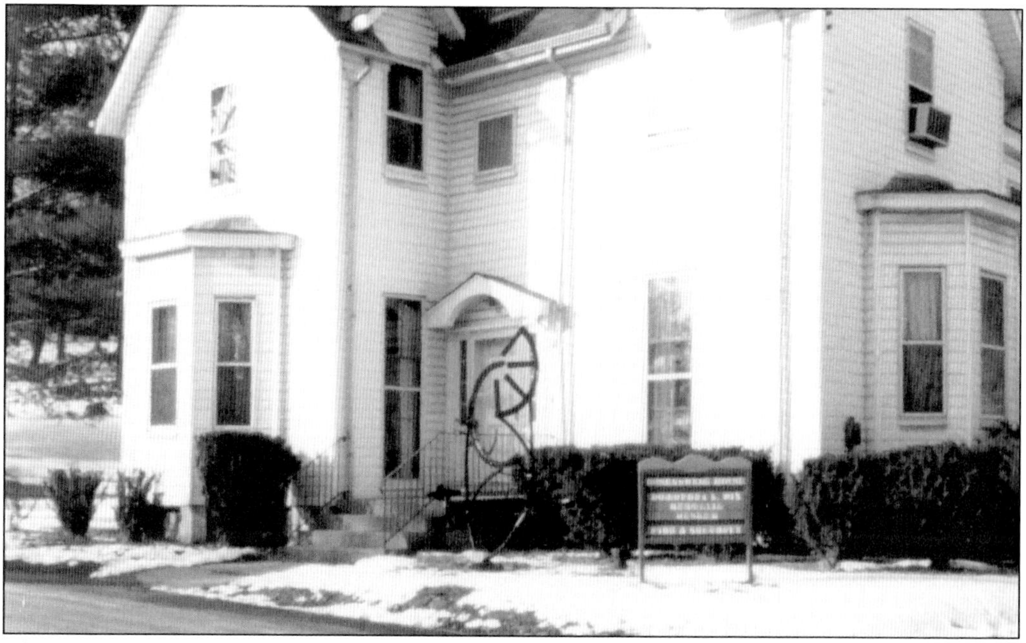

The Rosenzweig House, also known as the Reed House, was the residence of the superintendent. It was built in 1877 and was renovated in 1946, when an addition and aluminum siding were installed. Later the building was used for a small museum and security purposes. After Dixmont closed and ownership was transferred to the Stroyne family, the house was used as a guardhouse to protect the property from vandals. (Courtesy Tracy Ferguson.)

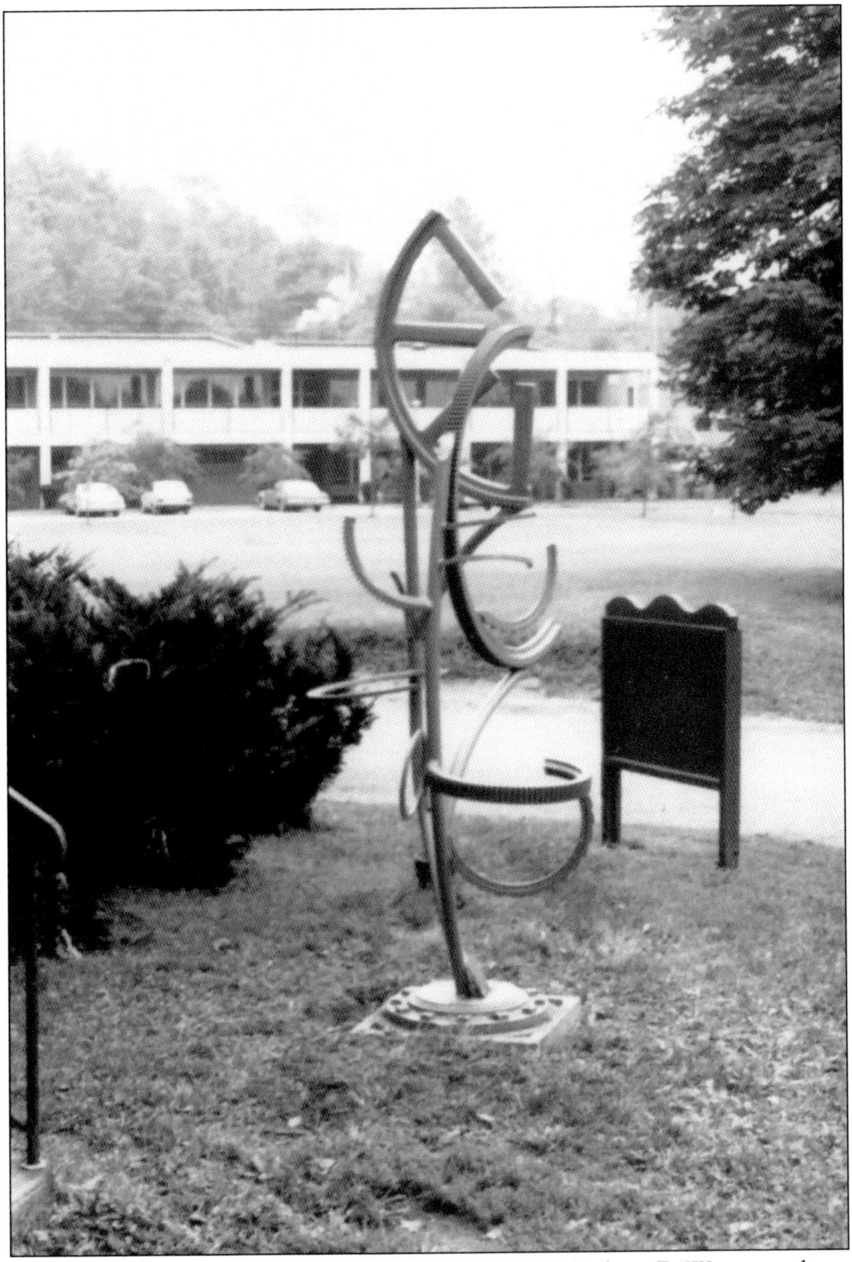

The Vital Balance was a sculpture borne of the tenure of Dr. Robert E. Weimer, who advocated removal of the bars from the windows of Dixmont State Hospital. The metal was used to create the sculpture. The title comes from a book penned by Dr. Karl Menninger, of whose work Dr. Weimer was obviously influenced by. "The critical functioning of ones personality between mental health (functioning) on one hand and emotional and mental problems on the other (dysfunction) is in each of us a matter of a 'Vital Balance,'" Dr. Weimer wrote to his staff in August 1967. "[Menninger] dispenses with meaningless labels and substitutes a concept where disturbed human behavior are but stages in a single, reversible process." Prior to its outdoor mounting in front of the Rosenzweig House, *The Vital Balance* was displayed in the entranceway of Reed Hall. (Courtesy Tracy Ferguson.)

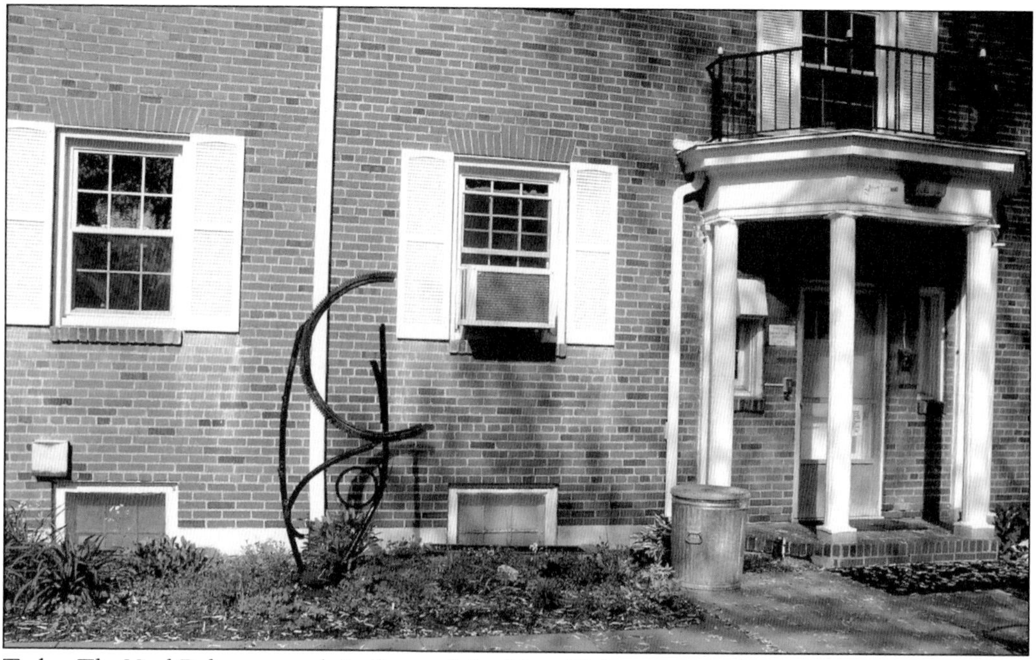

Today *The Vital Balance* stands in front of the Mary T. Summers Volunteer Center at Mayview State Hospital, where new patients and staff can admire it. Based on the writings of Dr. Karl Menninger, the sculpture represents the balance of mental functioning. According to Menninger, there were five mental dysfunctions, or imbalances: simple nervous, neurotic syndromes and personalities, naked aggression, psychoses, and malignant anxiety and depression that often led to suicide.

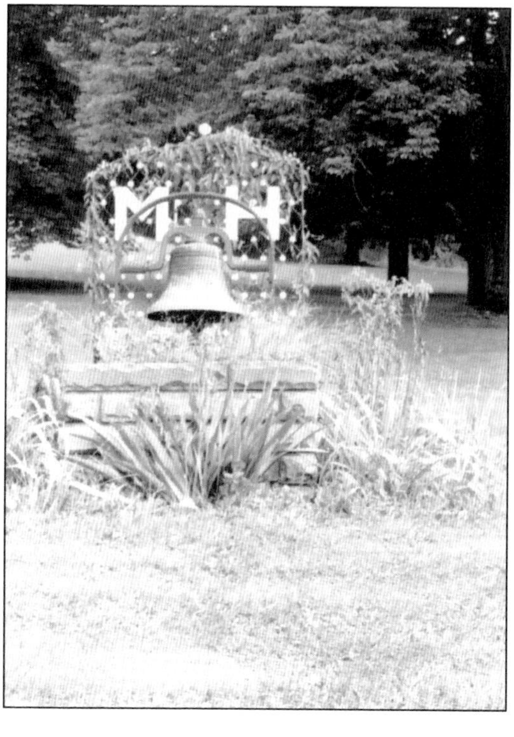

The *M* and *H* on this bell at Dixmont stood for mental health. Known as the "Ring the Bell for Mental Health" planter, the planter was made from the base of an antique treadle Singer sewing machine used by patients. It was designed by R. E. Finkler, the canteen manager. Ken Viney, Dixmont's institutional maintenance superintendent, helped create the final work. It was displayed in the lobby of Reed Hall during Mental Health Week 1971 before being moved outside. Tracy Ferguson, daughter of Dr. Robert Weimer, recounted a story of a patient at Dixmont who had the initials *M* and *H* in her name. The patient believed the bell to be hers. In 1976, the bell was painted red, white, and blue in honor of the bicentennial. (Courtesy Tracy Ferguson.)

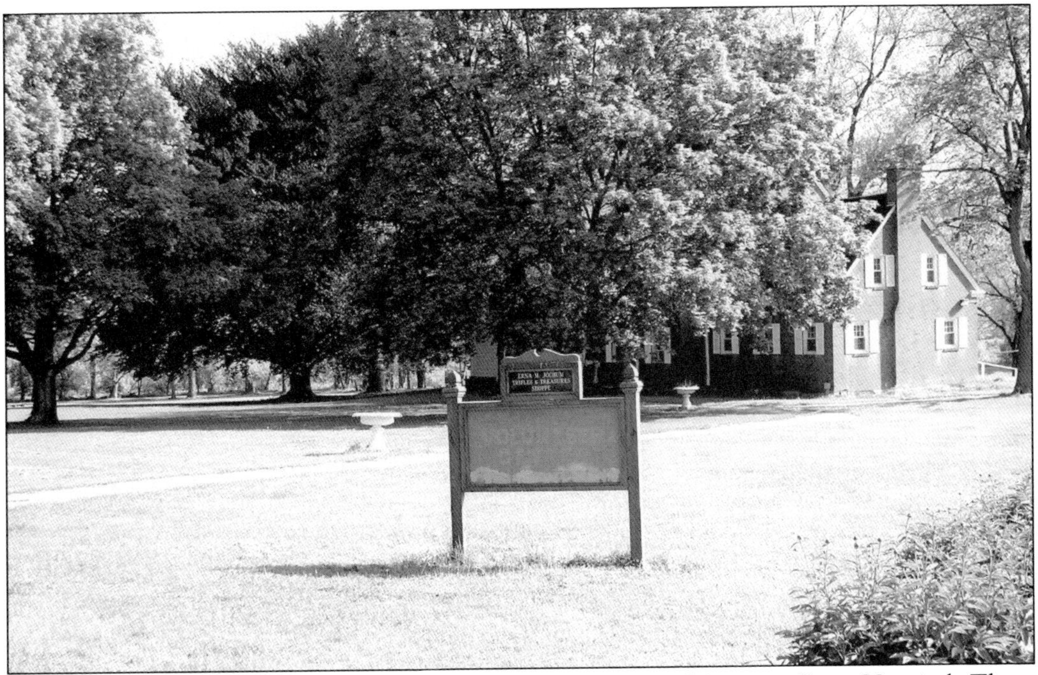

Not only antique furniture and artifacts found their way to Mayview State Hospital. These cement urns were lawn features at Dixmont before they became part of the landscape in front of the Erna M. Jochm Trifles and Treasures Shoppe at Mayview.

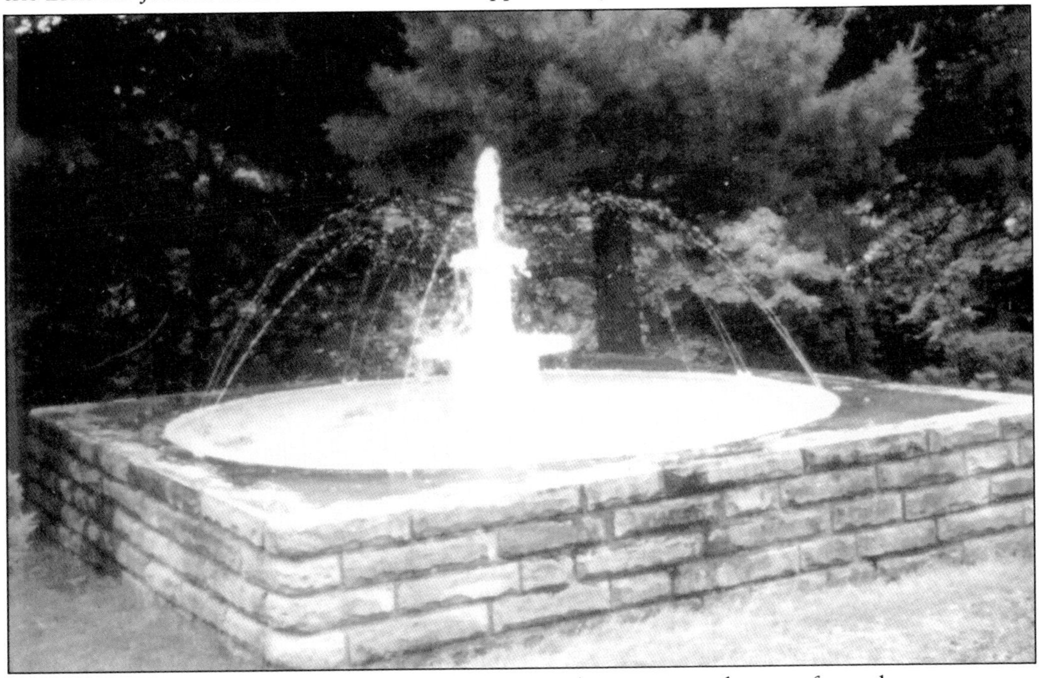

Part of Dixmont's landscape was this fountain, which was situated across from the entrance to Reed Hall. It was constructed in 1876. Dixmont also had a small religious shrine, a host of park benches, and other features to break up the landscape and create a parklike setting for patients. (Courtesy Tracy Ferguson.)

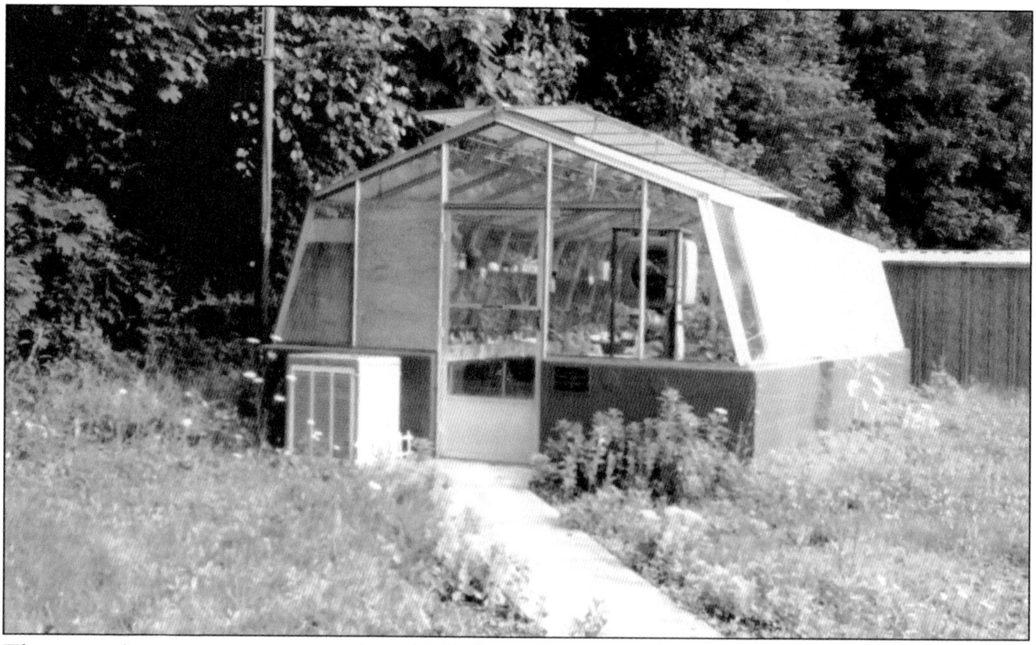

This greenhouse was constructed in 1973 through a grant from the Linke Fund, overseen by the Pittsburgh Foundation. By this point, the original Phipps greenhouse was long gone. This small replacement allowed patients to return to the original vision of Dr. Joseph Allison Reed by allowing them to beautify their surroundings with flowers of their own growing. Some of the first things planted were leeks, carnations, and tomatoes. Patients also started a tree farm of coleuses. (Courtesy Tracy Ferguson.)

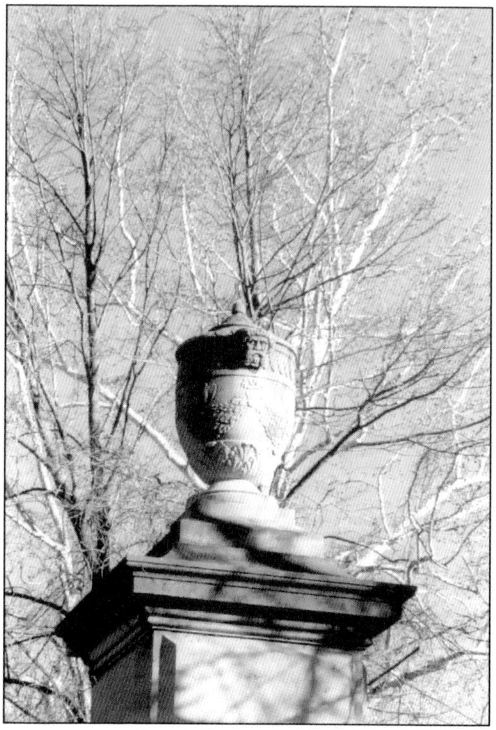

Two finial urns sat atop a pair of concrete pillars along the entranceway to Dixmont at the end of Huntington Avenue. At one time, the gateway was called the Reed Memorial Gate, funded by James H. Reed, grandson of Joseph Allison Reed. Shortly after the Stroyne family bought the property, the pillars were removed and sold to an antiques collector in Chicago for about $1,000 each. Ralph Stroyne said he could not sell them for much because they were damaged.

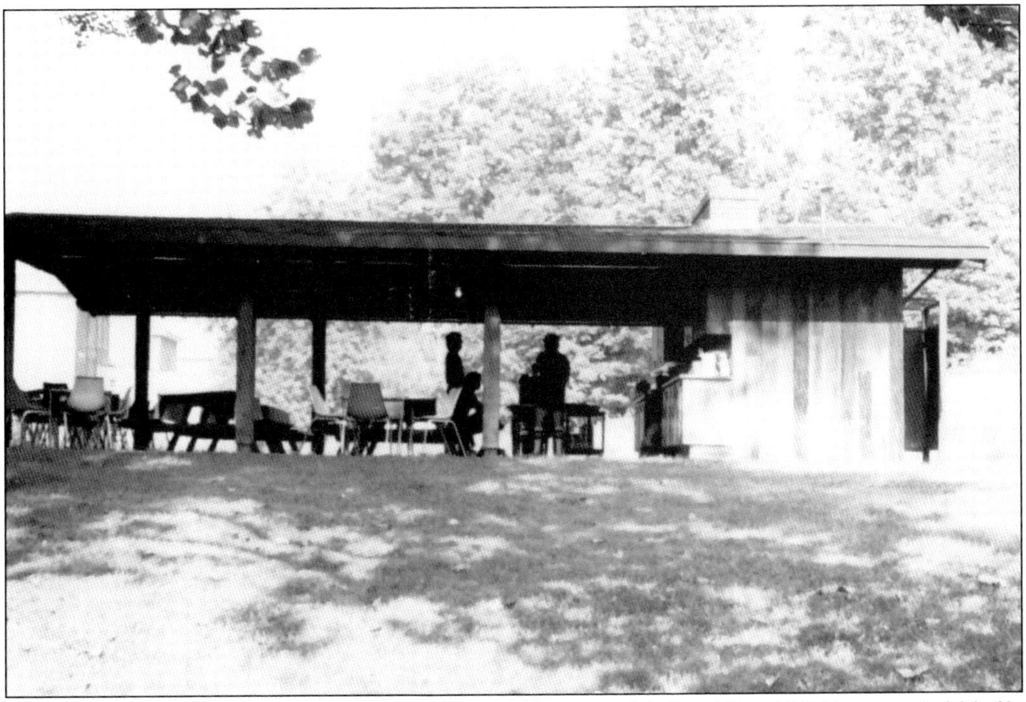

There were two picnic pavilions at Dixmont, each situated behind Reed Hall on graded bluffs. They had restrooms, running water, and electricity. The areas were excellent places for patients to catch some air and smoke. This pavilion was constructed with $1,600 worth of funding from the Rachelwood Foundation in 1969.

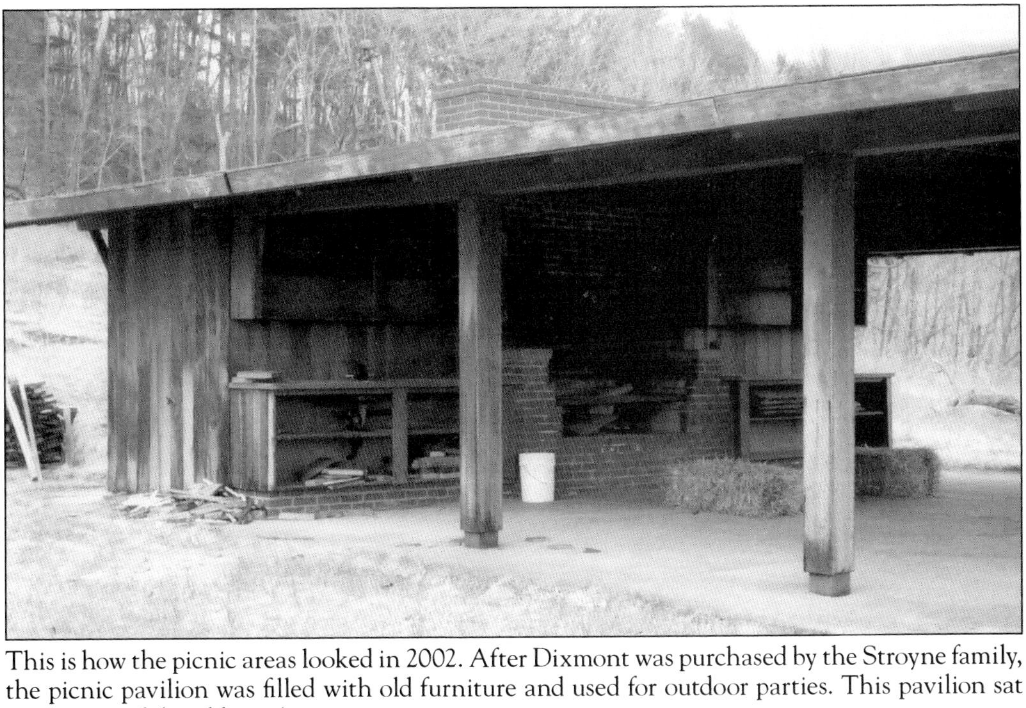

This is how the picnic areas looked in 2002. After Dixmont was purchased by the Stroyne family, the picnic pavilion was filled with old furniture and used for outdoor parties. This pavilion sat on the site of the old men's annex.

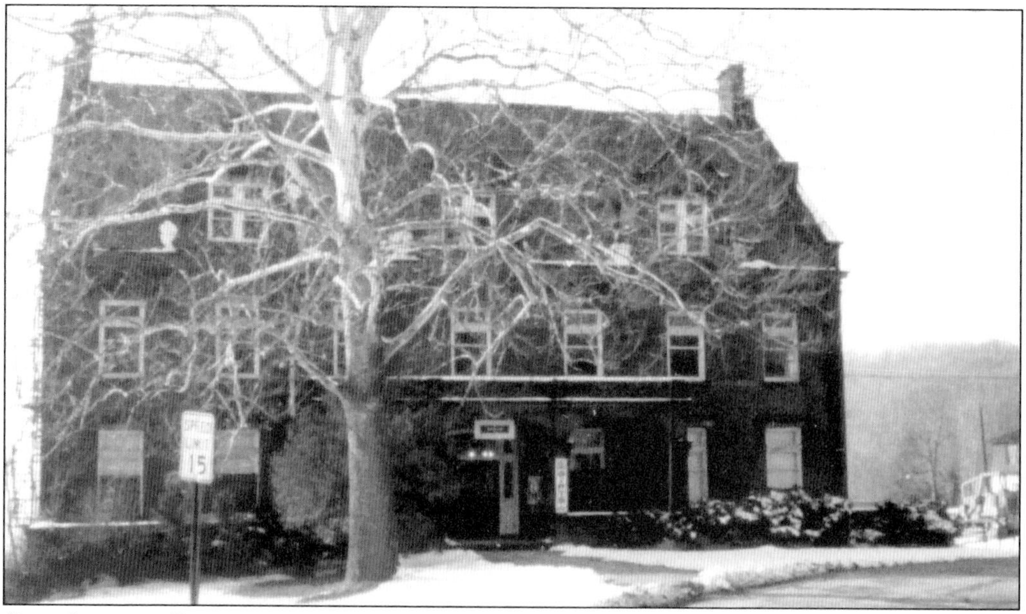

Once home to Dixmont's nurses, the nurses' dormitory later became renamed the Dixieland Canteen and was informally called the Dixie Duds, the name of the small second-hand clothing shop it housed. It served as a small general shop for patients and staff. It also was the base of the volunteer department.

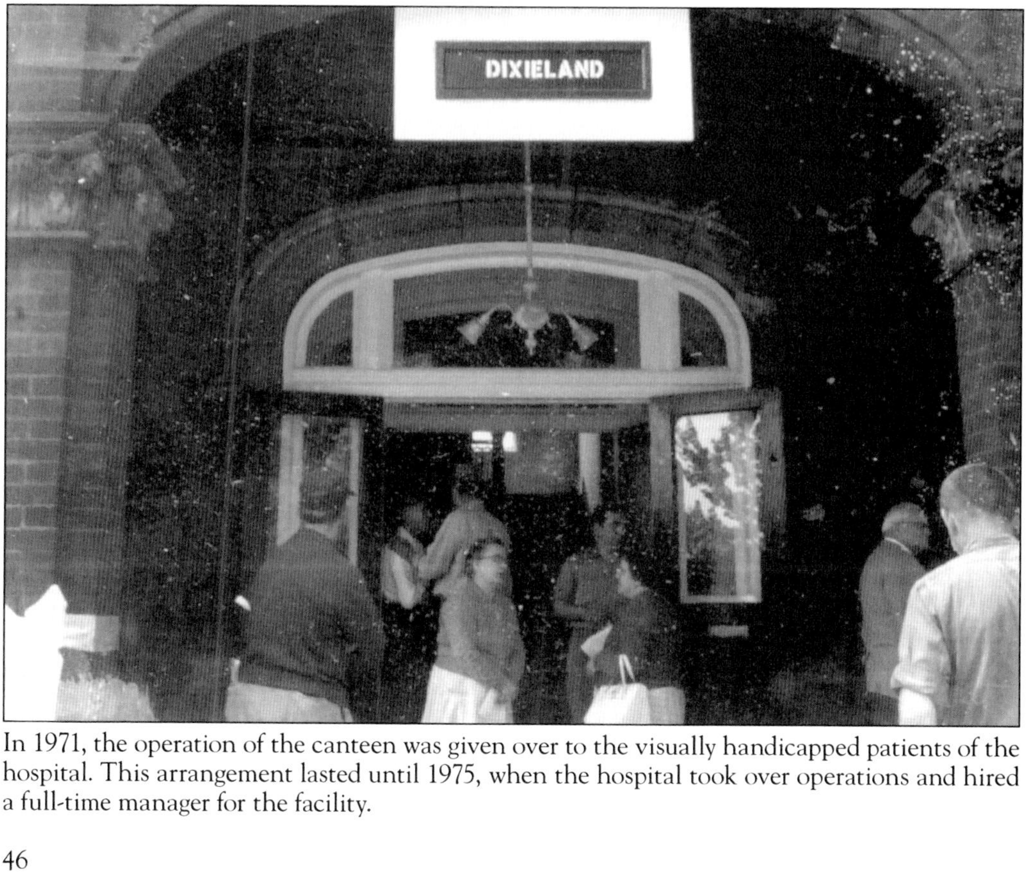

In 1971, the operation of the canteen was given over to the visually handicapped patients of the hospital. This arrangement lasted until 1975, when the hospital took over operations and hired a full-time manager for the facility.

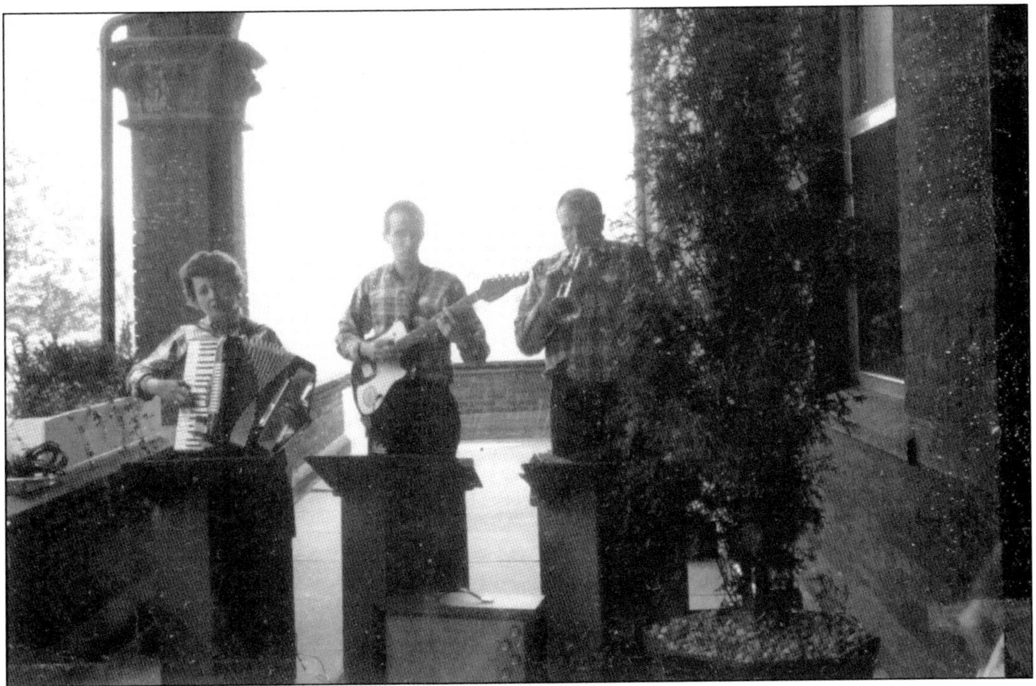

When the Dixieland Canteen reopened, there was a celebration complete with a three-piece Dixieland jazz band. Here the band, made up of Joann Johnston, a recreation employee, and two patients, Ralph (center) and Leonard, plays on the porch. Dixmont was a hospital, but it was also a home. Many patients lent their talents to the hospital.

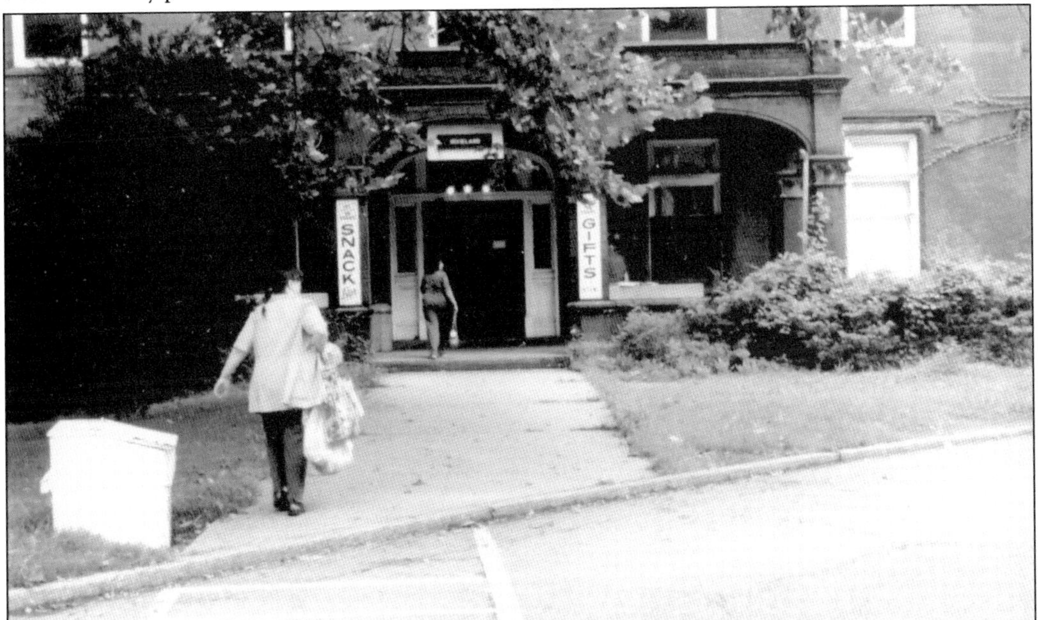

The Dixieland Canteen looked to be much more than it was. In reality, the top floors of the building were closed, leaving essentially a one-story operation in a three-story structure. There was a sewing room situated in the rear of the building.

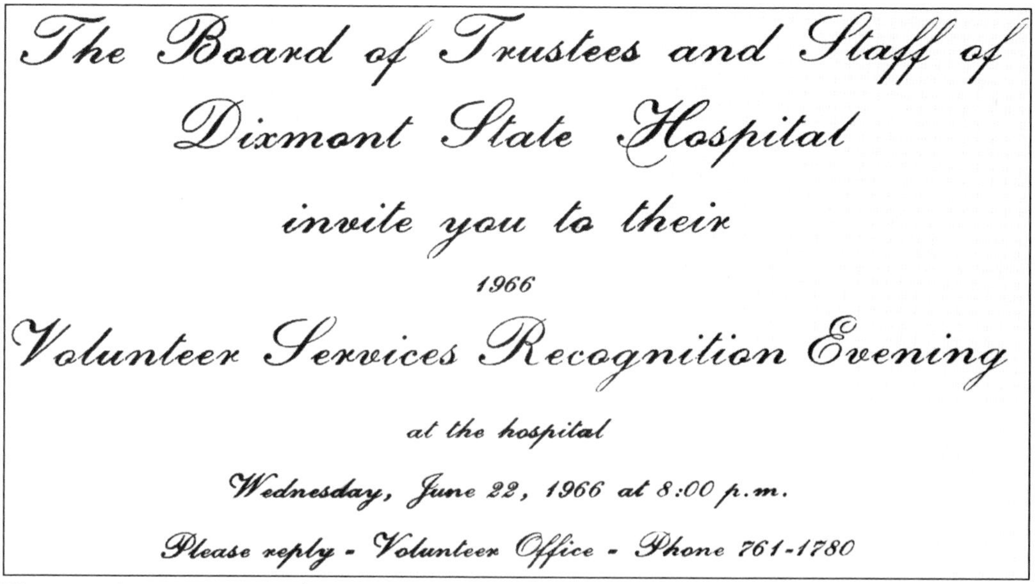

The Board of Trustees and Staff of
Dixmont State Hospital
invite you to their
1966
Volunteer Services Recognition Evening
at the hospital
Wednesday, June 22, 1966 at 8:00 p.m.
Please reply - Volunteer Office - Phone 761-1780

This was the invitation to the June 22, 1966, Volunteer Services recognition party. Dr. Robert Weimer's official creed for the hospital was Francis Peabody's 1927 statement: "The secret of the care of the patient is in the caring for the patient." Recognized for their total care for the patients of Dixmont, the volunteers were formally recognized at dinners such as this and in the staff and volunteer newsletters.

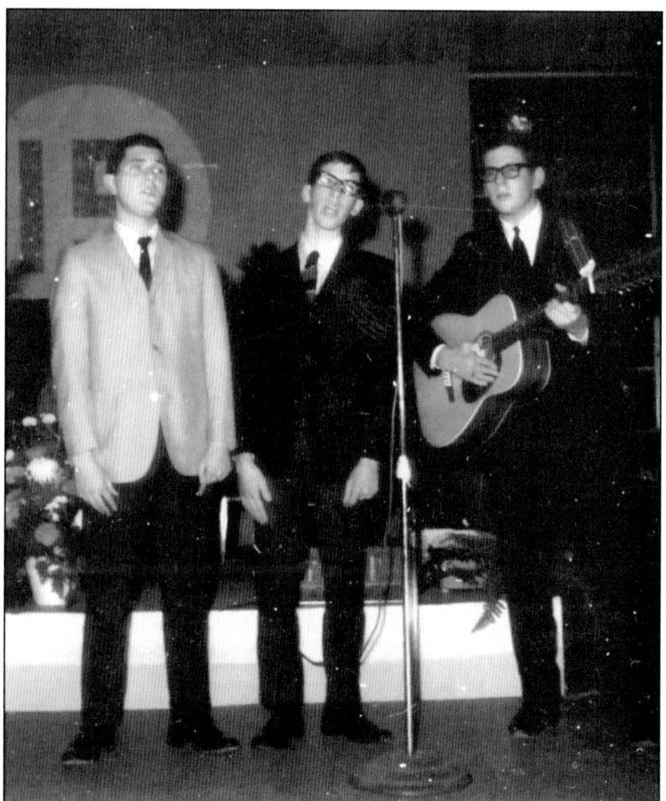

Throughout the years, volunteer musicians entertained the patients with performances at Dixmont. For a long stretch of time, the Belairs played music at the hospital every Wednesday evening. Here musicians play for the volunteer recognition party.

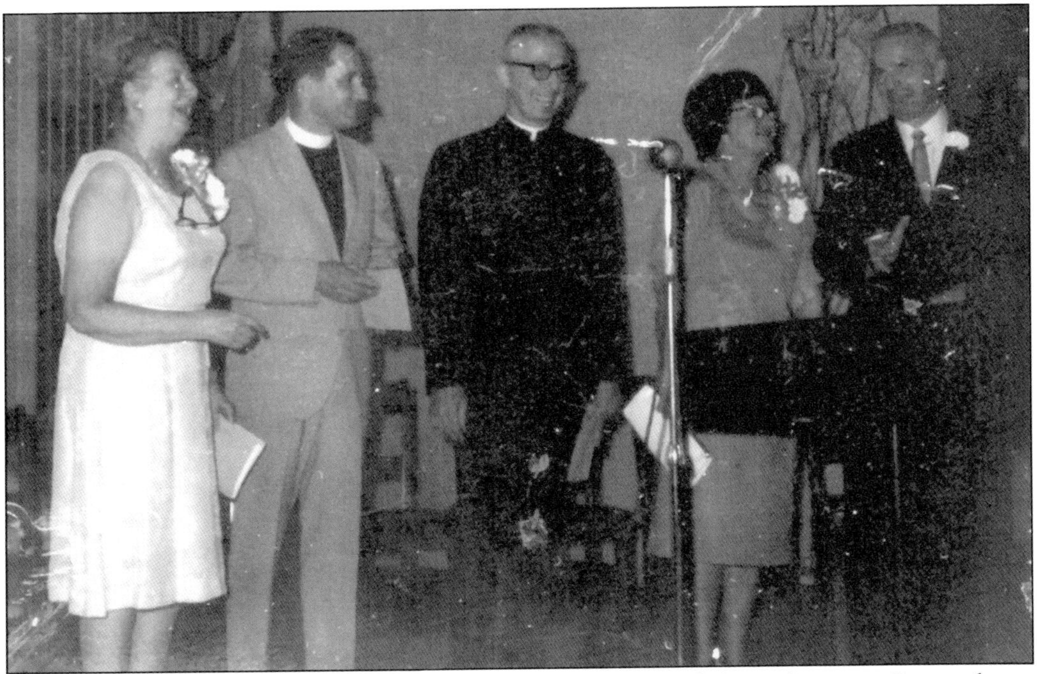

In this photograph, hospital officials recognize the works of the volunteers. Pictured are, from left to right, Clara Walsh, volunteer coordinator; two unidentified clergymen; Margaret McBride, member of the board of trustees; and Dr. Robert Weimer, superintendent. Dixmont had a revolving relationship with many local churches and synagogues from which religious representatives would come to the hospital to perform ceremonies throughout the year.

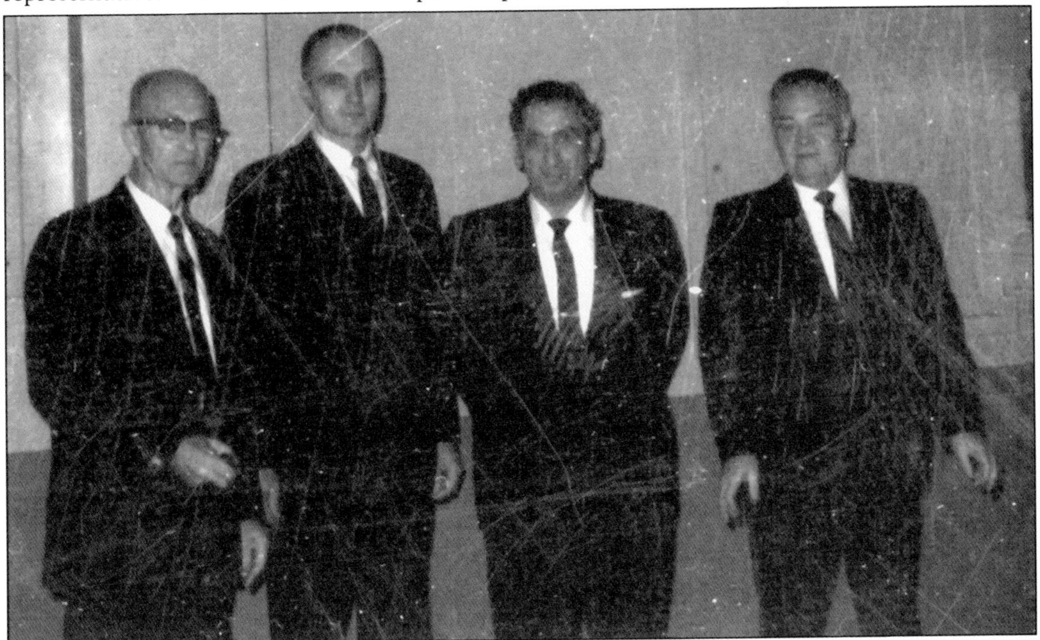

From left to right, Henry Woodburn (maintenance department), unidentified, Alex Quattrochi, and another unidentified man gather for a photograph at the Volunteer Services recognition dinner. (Courtesy Helen Wolf.)

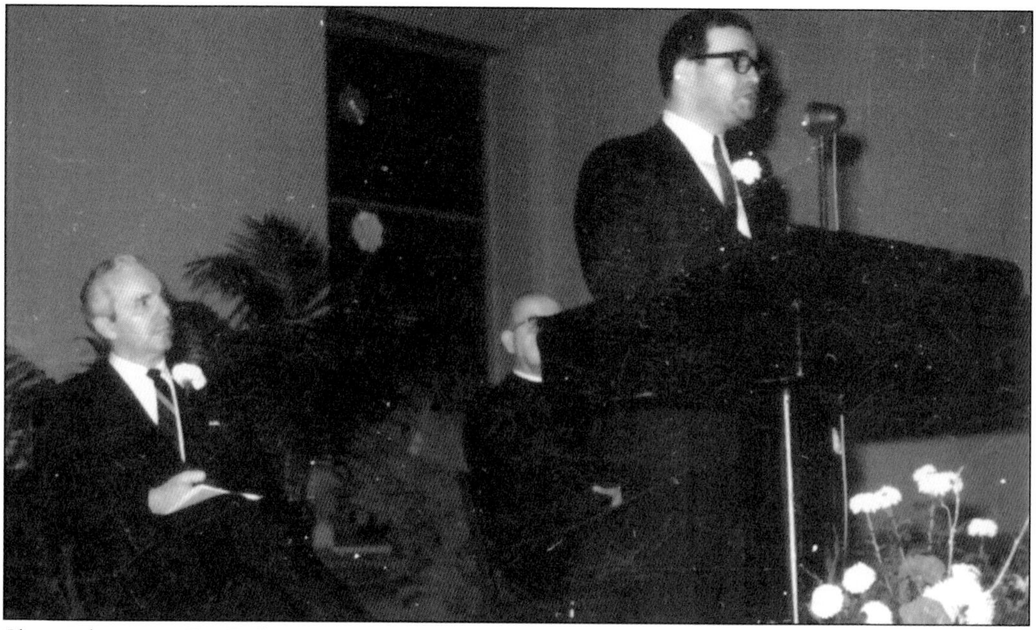

Shown here are Dr. Robert Weimer, seated, and Dr. Leroy R. Weiner, a longtime member of the Dixmont Board of Trustees. Dr. Weiner, a former president of the board for Dixmont, died of cancer in Greenwich, Connecticut, on September 24, 1984. He was the 1961 Pennsylvania NAACP human rights award recipient and treasurer of the Pennsylvania Equal Rights Council. (Courtesy Helen Wolf.)

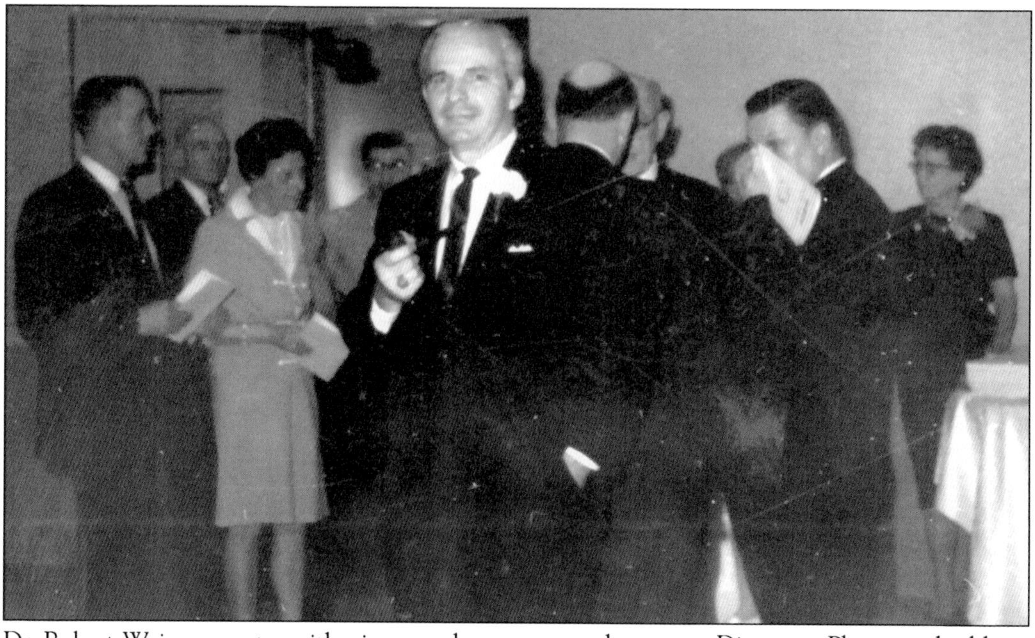

Dr. Robert Weimer, center with pipe, was key to many changes at Dixmont. Photographed here during the hospital's first employee recognition night, Dr. Weimer was an instrument of change for Dixmont. He hired the first fire marshal and librarian for the hospital. The historical committee was founded under his tenure. Perhaps most importantly, Dr. Weimer was known for removing the bars from the windows of Dixmont and for starting a deaf unit. (Courtesy Helen Wolf.)

Social services director Anne Scholtze serves up some punch at the Volunteer Services recognition dinner in November 1959. Dedication to the patient was the soul of Dixmont, but the volunteers were the heart. Volunteers provided thousands of hours of donated time each year, according to reports. (Courtesy Helen Wolf.)

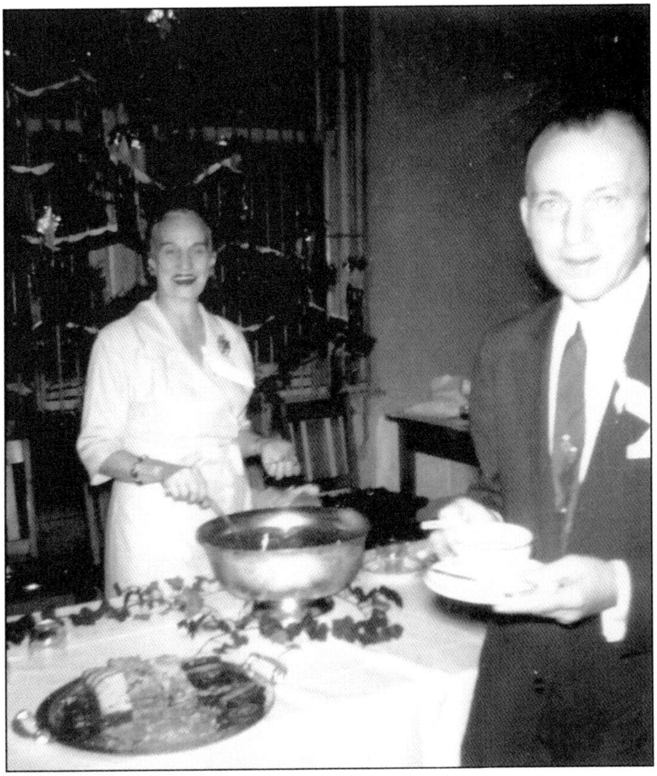

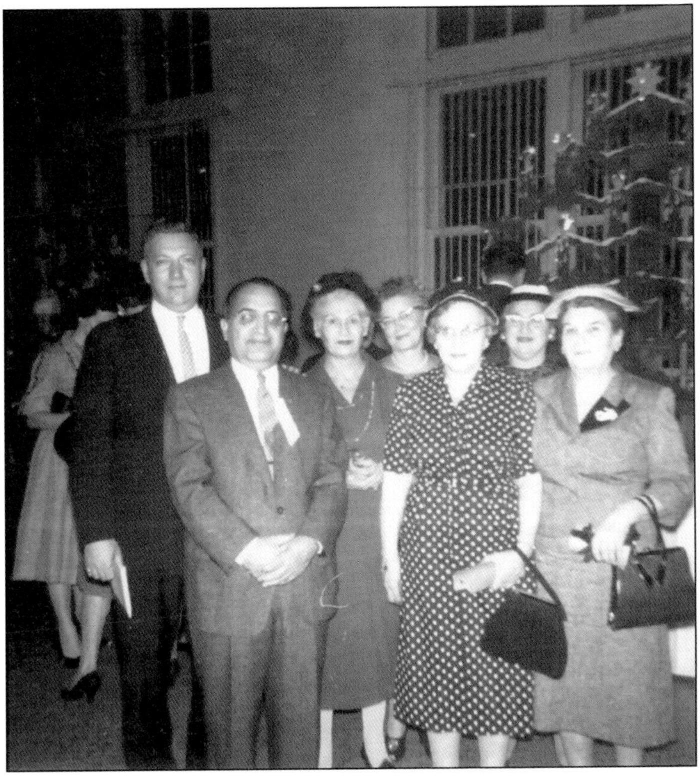

The cavernous halls in the dietary building were used frequently for large get togethers and functions. Here Dr. Joseph Cammarata, second from the left, stands with an unidentified group at a Christmas function. Wards would decorate for holidays, and oftentimes there were contests for the best decorated ward. The winners were written up in the staff newsletter. (Courtesy Helen Wolf.)

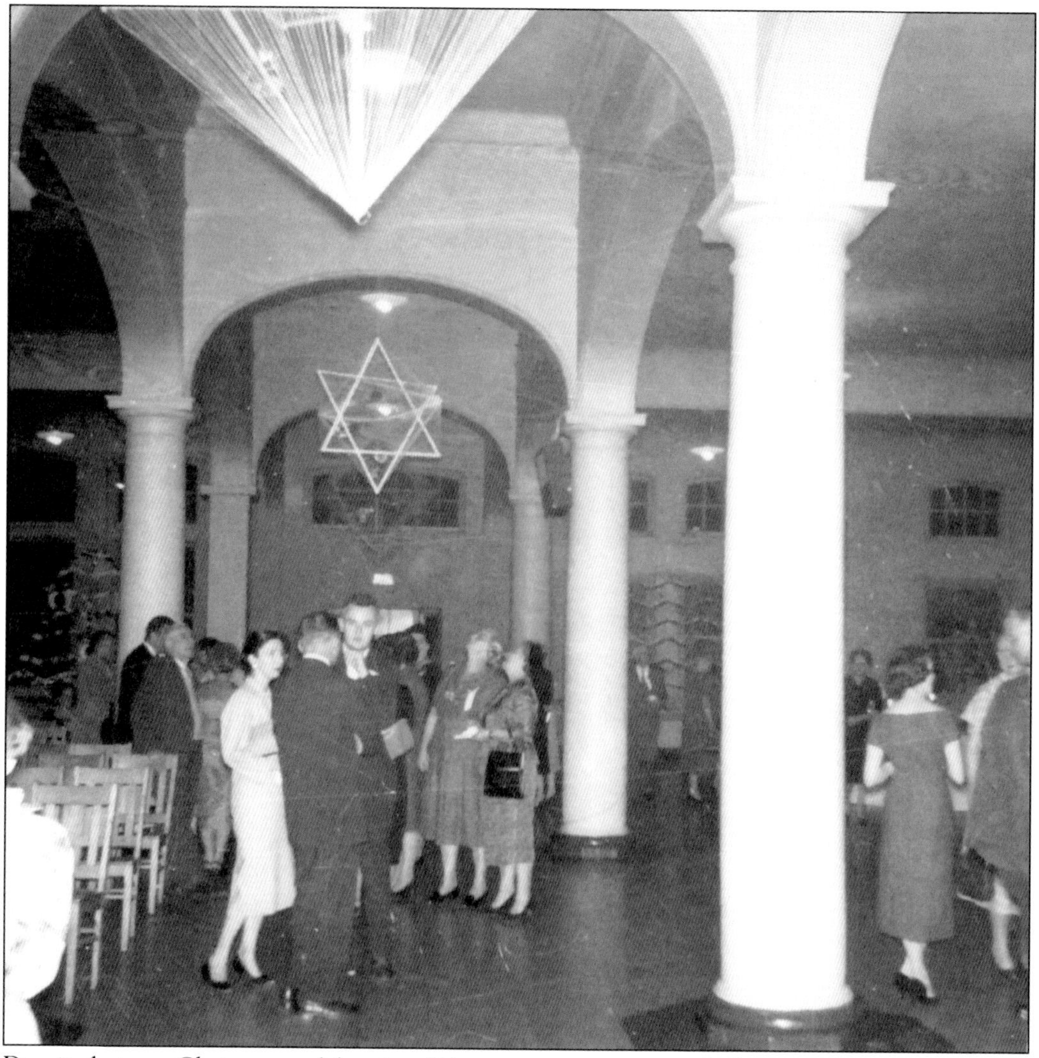

Despite being a Christmas celebration, Dixmont patients were of all nationalities and religious denominations. Holidays were celebrated by all. Pictured here is a Star of David display in the dietary building in 1959. During these holidays, patients routinely received stockings and cigarettes as gifts by Santas and "Santa Belles." (Courtesy Helen Wolf.)

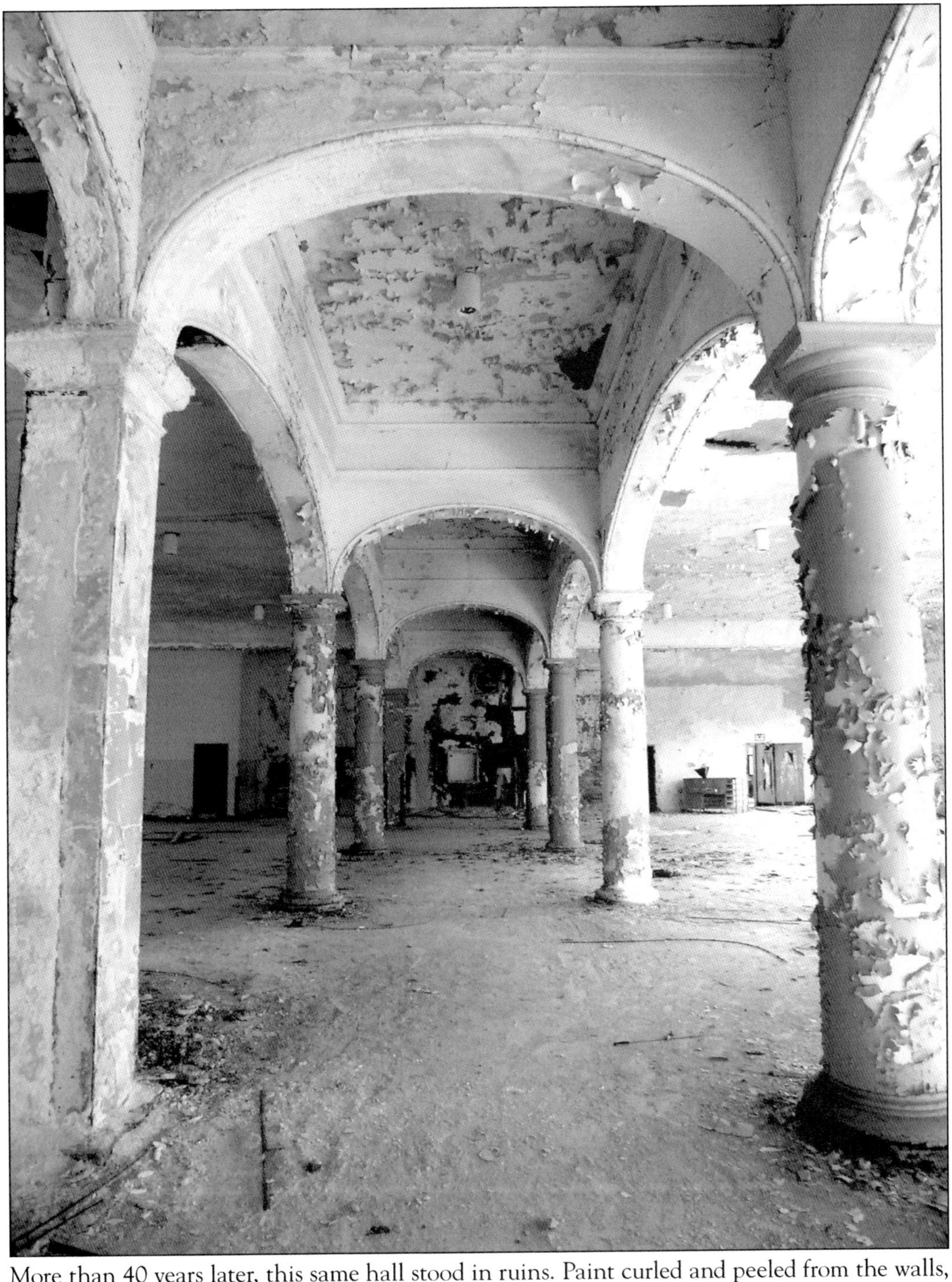

More than 40 years later, this same hall stood in ruins. Paint curled and peeled from the walls, and new paint in the form of graffiti was applied. This space, which once held celebrations by staff and patients, became a favorite spot for filming amateur horror movies and for hosting ghost hunts.

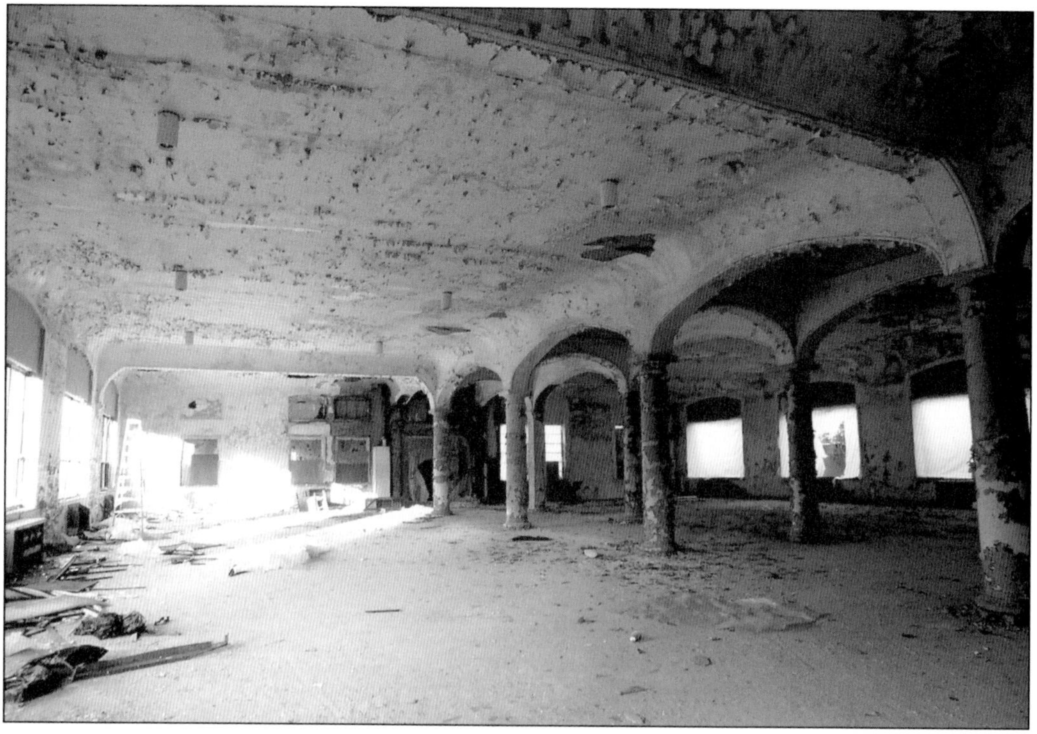

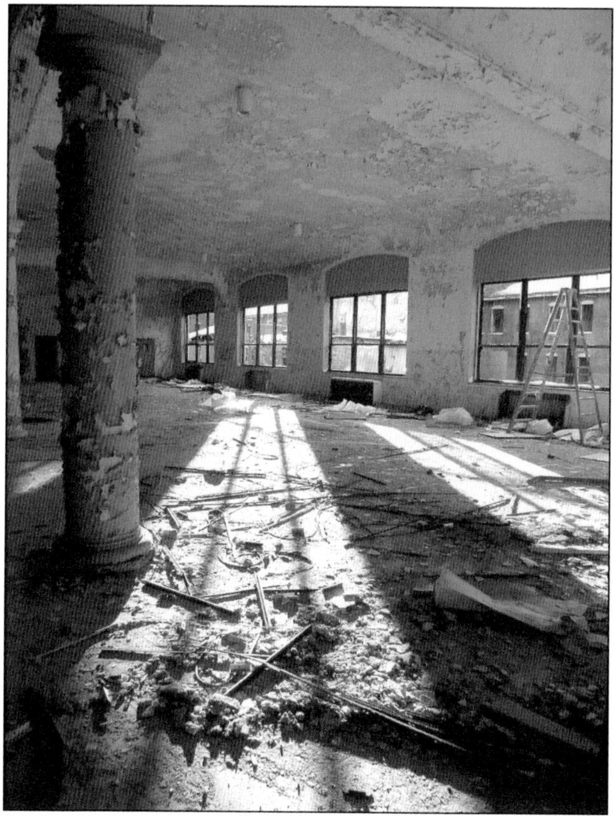

Inside the second floor of the dietary building were two large dining halls with vaulted ceilings. These areas served as dining areas and space to hold events. In 1968, the Beaver Unit dining area was designated as the primary dining hall, and the Lawrence Unit dining area became a recreational area. A small stage was installed, and performances were put on to entertain the patients and staff.

Two

Celebration Day

Dixmont State Hospital, by virtue of its location, was both in the middle of a busy Pittsburgh thoroughfare and hidden from view. The hospital was known by its landmark smokestack attached to the boiler house, the only structure that could be clearly seen from Route 65. Despite that, Dixmont was a bustling miniature community. The adopted creed of the hospital became, "The secret of the care of the patient is in caring for the patient." So many of the hospital activities were focused on keeping the patients occupied that there was no trouble finding people to do the necessary work to keep Dixmont beautified and current. Holiday decorations were made by occupational therapy patients and holiday carols sung by a patient chorus. When the hospital first started, patients tended gardens, herded livestock, and made crafts to decorate their surroundings. Dr. Joseph Allison Reed strongly believed that the beautification of the hospital and its grounds was key to patient recuperation.

This belief stuck with the hospital. And while the state cut Dixmont's budget year after year, staff and volunteers strived to maintain a quality of life for the patients that was unaffected by tightening purse strings.

In 1966, when Dr. Robert Weimer took the helm as the fourth superintendent in Dixmont's history, the period informally referred to as "Dixmont's Renaissance" began. Bars were removed from the hospital, and the metal was used to make sculptures and furniture. Picnic areas were added through foundation funding. A new greenhouse was added, also through foundation funding. Dr. Weimer and his staff were apparent masters of working with what they had to work with while maintaining the dignity and well being of those entrusted to their care.

It was a period of time that was to be celebrated, and Dixmont had plenty of celebrations. One of the most notable celebrations was the outdoor festivals or carnivals created by staff and volunteers for the patients. These grand endeavors included booths for food and games of chance, floats, and grandiose constructions. While staff participated in the event as well as put it on, the events were ultimately for the patients, who were part of this great family of healing.

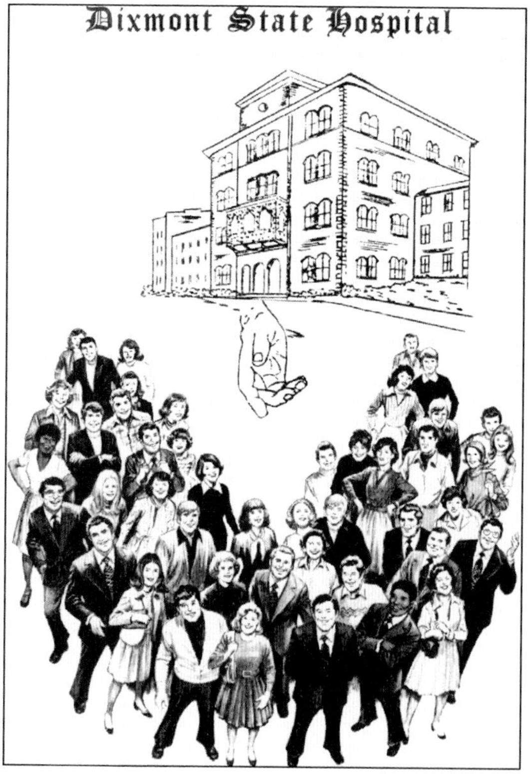

During the tenure of Dr. Robert Weimer, the period known as the Dixmont Renaissance occurred. It was a period of openness at Dixmont when the bars came off the windows and the hospital functioned as an active member of the community. Here is a cover from a program for an open house at Dixmont, which was held Tuesday and Wednesday, May 13 and 14, 1975. The cover was designed by Ruth Grimsley and depicts Dixmont's "appeal to the people of the community for their Helping Hand Towards Good Mental Health." (Courtesy Leroy Egan.)

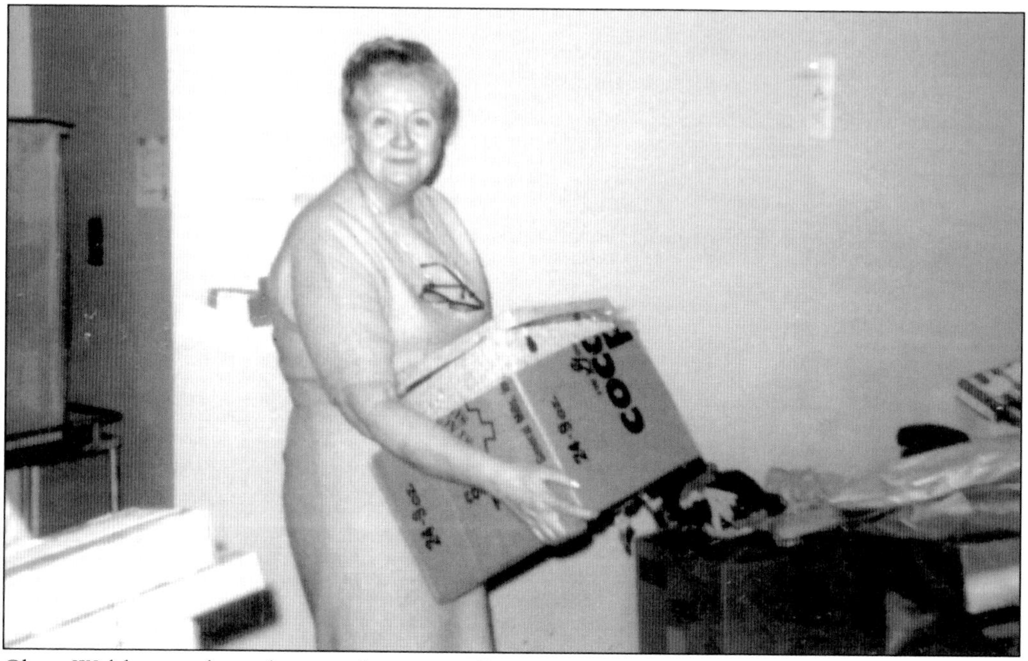

Clara Walsh was the volunteer director at Dixmont State Hospital. She began her career at Dixmont in the early 1960s and was revered by her volunteers. Walsh was instrumental in the many functions and celebrations at Dixmont. She later retired from the hospital and is now deceased. (Courtesy Helen Wolf.)

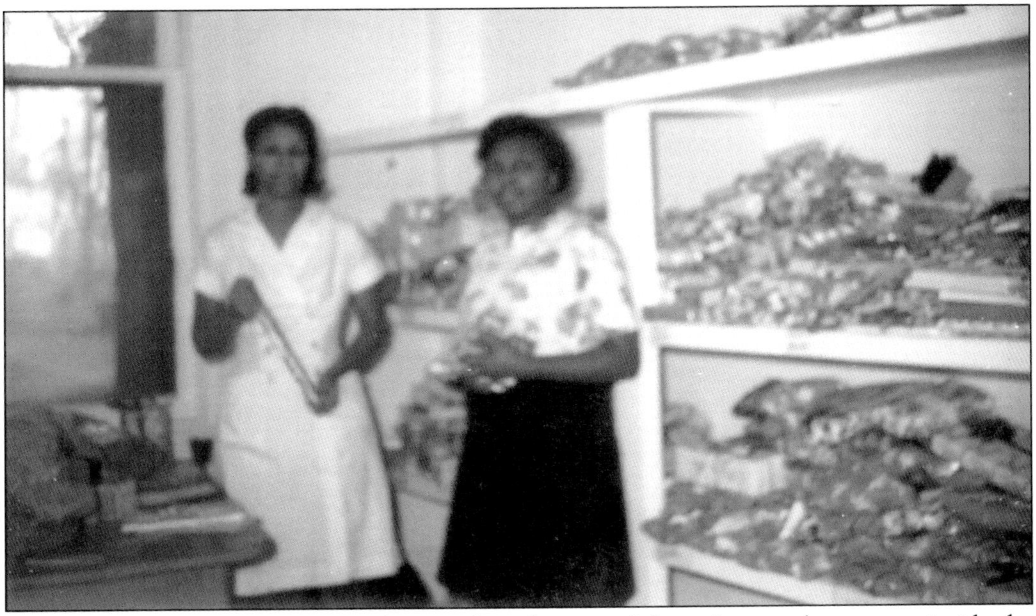

These unidentified nurses are standing in the gift room of the volunteer department inside the Dixieland Canteen building—formerly the nurses' dormitory. Staff and volunteers would wrap and disseminate the gifts to the patients on holidays and special occasions so that everyone received something special. Gifts were considered to be especially important because they were tangible evidence of caring. Many patients received no visitors, and gifts came only from volunteer efforts. (Courtesy Helen Wolf.)

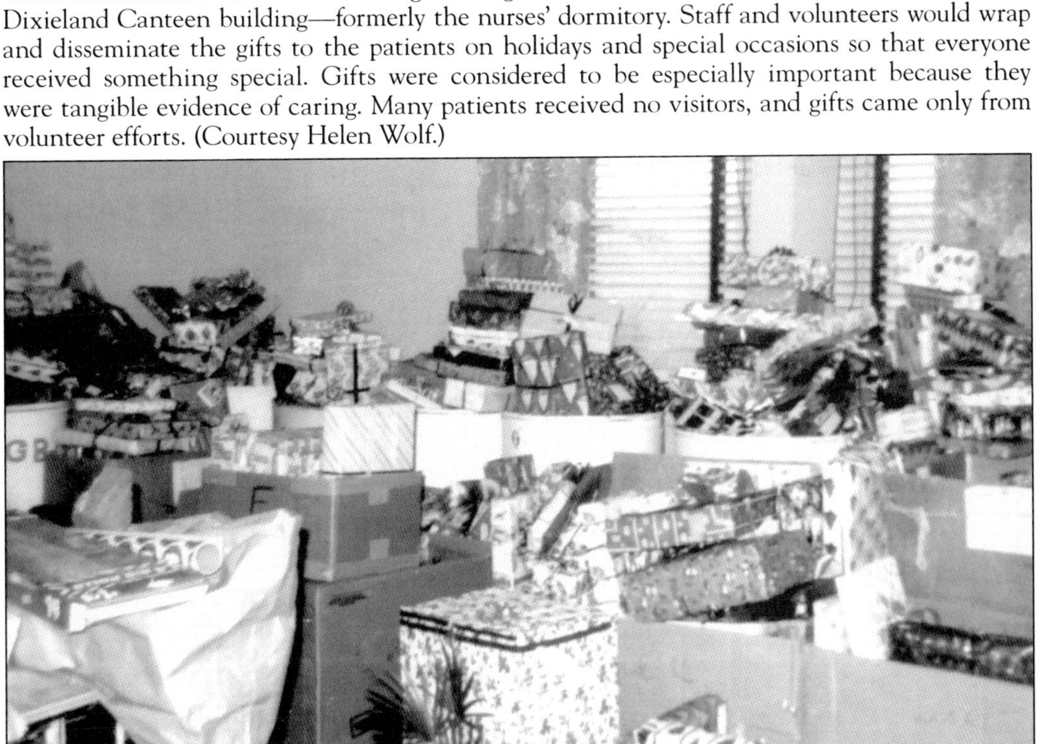

The gift room was overflowing with generous donations from patient relatives, staff members, volunteers, and community groups. Holidays of all denominations were celebrated at Dixmont, as there were patients of all faiths living on the premises. Volunteers sorted and wrapped gifts for the patients. (Courtesy Helen Wolf.)

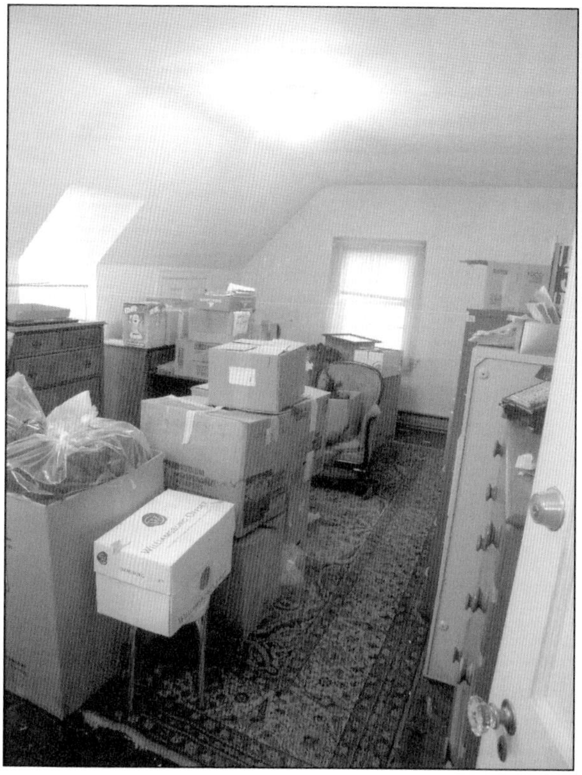

This room at Mayview State Hospital is on the top floor of the Mary T. Summers Volunteer Center and serves double duty both as a storage room for Dixmont photographs and antiques and as a gift room for storing donated gifts for Mayview's patient population. Summers was the first volunteer coordinator in the state and remained at Mayview throughout her career.

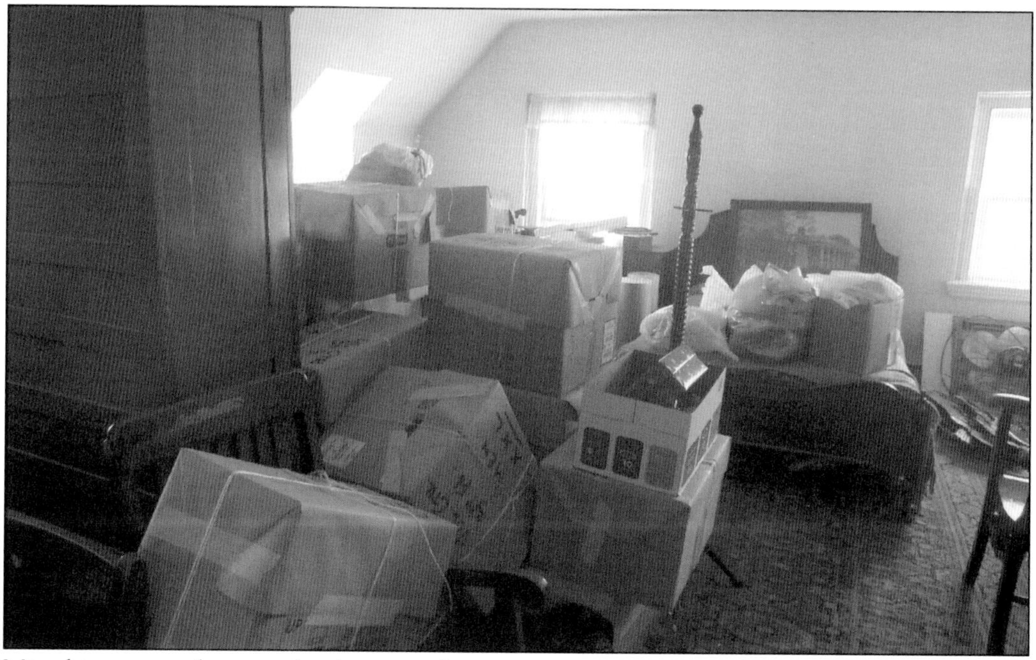

Mixed in among these randomly strewn boxes are vintage items such as an eyeglass fitting kit, photographs of the groundbreaking of Dixmont's Cammarata Building, furniture from Dixmont, and more. The top floor of this building also is home to "Mr. Bones," a human skeleton from Dixmont used for medical training purposes.

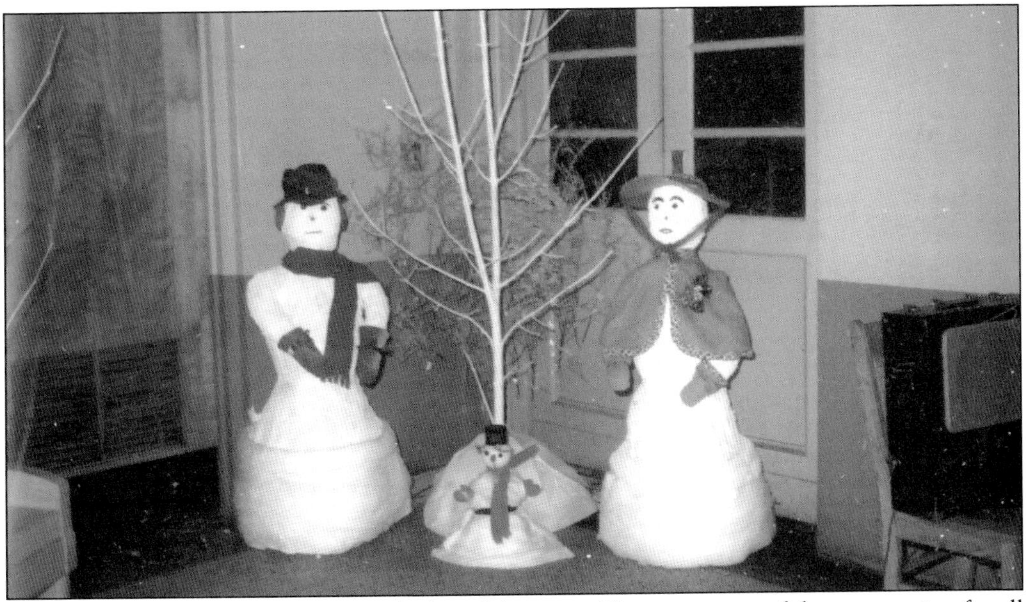

Patients were not just recipients of gifts for celebrations. They were part of the preparation for all of the events that were part of their home. Depicted here is a snowman family. While surviving Dixmont staff could not verify who made this display, consensus was that the display, like many others, was made in the occupational therapy department by patients. The occupational therapy department made many decorations for the hospital such as macramé plant hangers and displays of roses.

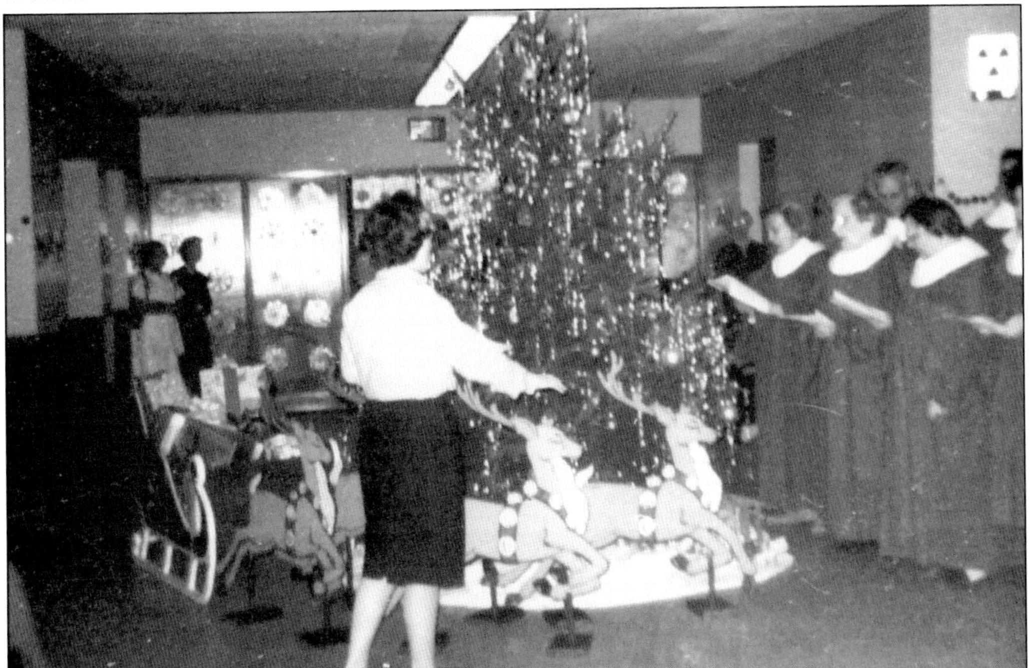

Once the displays were made and the tinsel hung, Christmas was celebrated as it would be in any other venue. Here Georgiana Buckwalter conducts the Dixmont Patient Chorus in Christmas carols. Buckwalter was the musical director at Dixmont. (Courtesy Helen Wolf.)

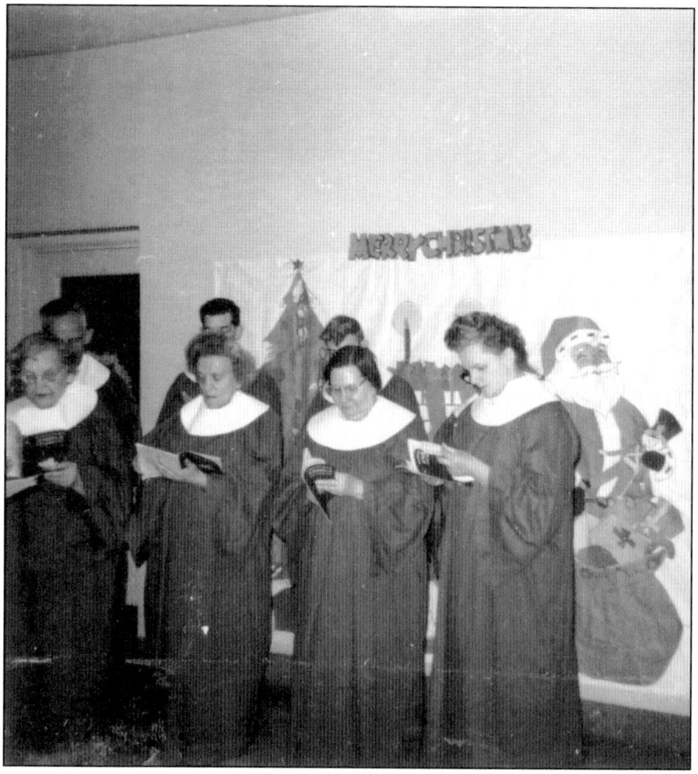

Here is another photograph of Dixmont's patient chorus celebrating Christmas. Dixmont also held an annual Halloween party and Monte Carlo night. Costumes for the Halloween parties were donated by groups, organizations, and individuals. (Courtesy Helen Wolf.)

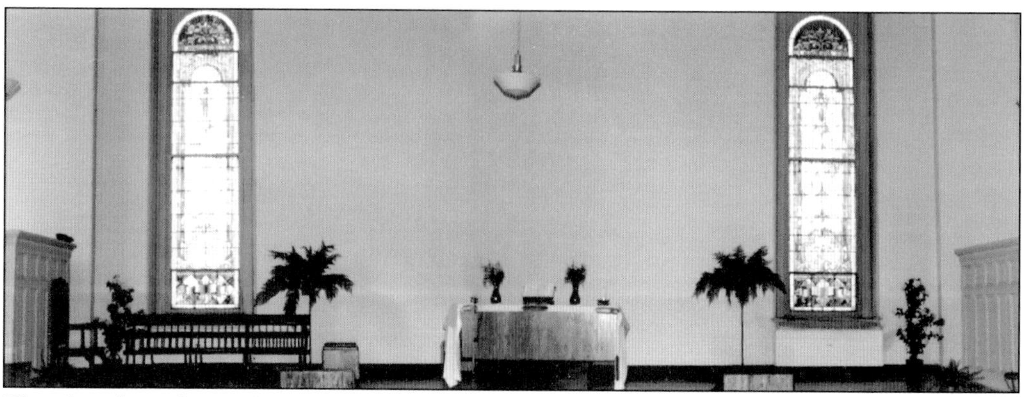

The chapel inside Reed Hall was a staple of Dixmont's operations. Located on the third floor, the chapel served as a nondenominational area for worship and lectures. It was complete with stained-glass windows designed and installed in 1859 by Yugoslavian craftsmen. They were covered with bars. Dixmont employed a staff reverend, and invited Jewish, Protestant, and Presbyterian ministers to celebrate services with patients. (Courtesy Tracy Ferguson.)

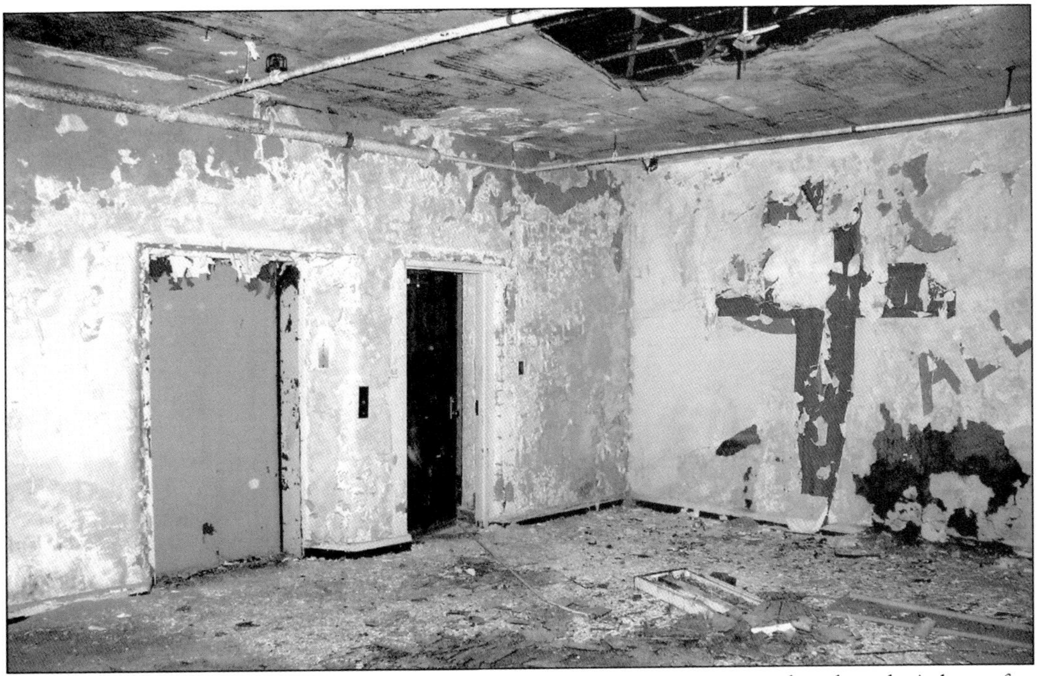

This rare view is on the third floor of Reed Hall at the entryway to the chapel. A large fire occurred in this area in 1995, resulting in the caved-in ceilings. The "Alleluia" mural can be seen on the far wall and is one of the many murals that staff painted throughout Dixmont.

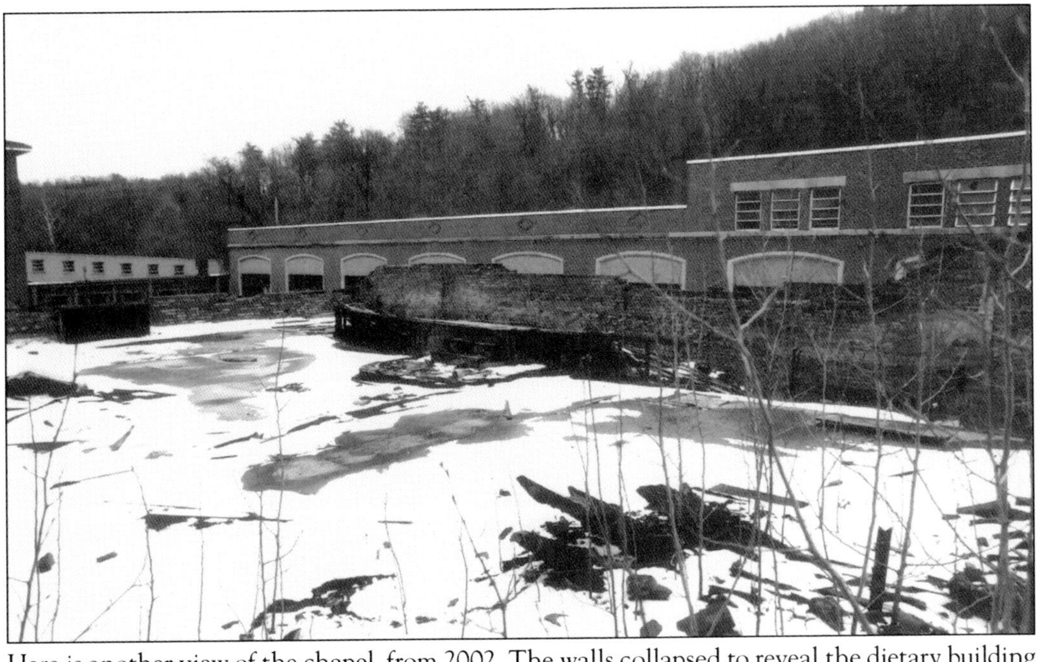

Here is another view of the chapel, from 2002. The walls collapsed to reveal the dietary building in the background. The remains of the alter can be seen arcing around the rear wall of the chapel. Over time, weeds, moss, and mold took over much of Dixmont, growing from crevasses that one would not normally expect them to grow from, such as the floor of the exposed chapel.

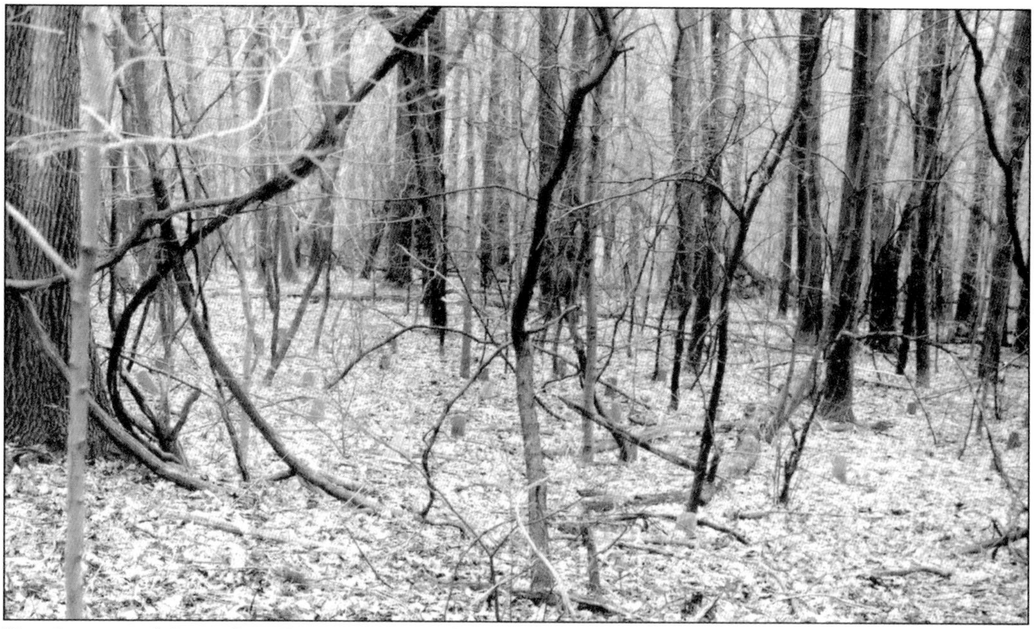

Death was celebrated at Dixmont as well. The property has a cemetery with an estimated 1,300 graves. This cemetery, which still is property of the Commonwealth of Pennsylvania, is in a state of severe neglect. The graves are simply numbered obelisks standing about two feet tall. The numbers correspond to a list of names that provide little detail as to who is buried in the cemetery.

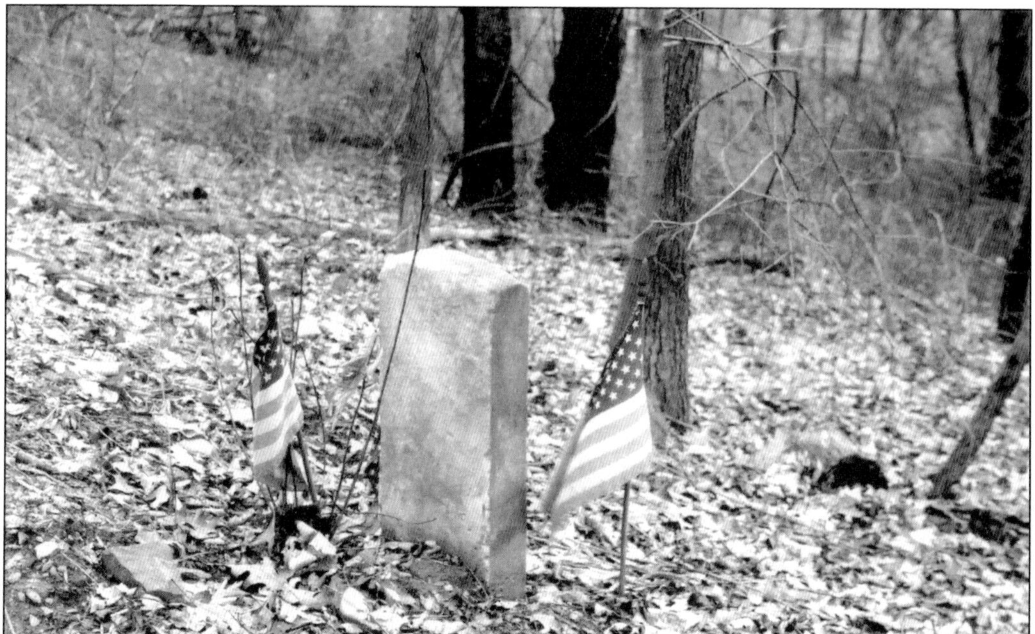

Despite the anonymity of those buried in Dixmont's cemetery, there are certain graves that stand out. These tend to be the graves of known war veterans. Dixmont opened its doors as a makeshift general services hospital during the Civil War. The veterans' graves are sometimes decorated by local residents on Memorial Day.

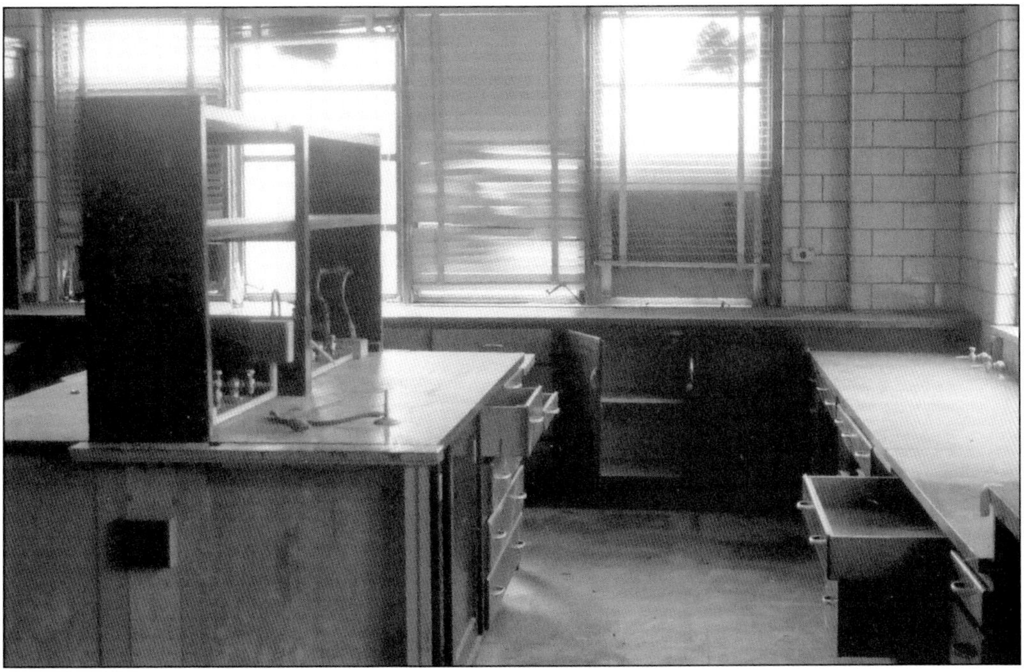

One of the more familiar sections of the Hutchinson Building is the laboratory, which was on the ground floor. Because of its location, the windows were easily broken out, and the laboratory was ransacked by vandals. This view faces Route 65, and gas nozzles and a Bunsen burner can be seen on the counters.

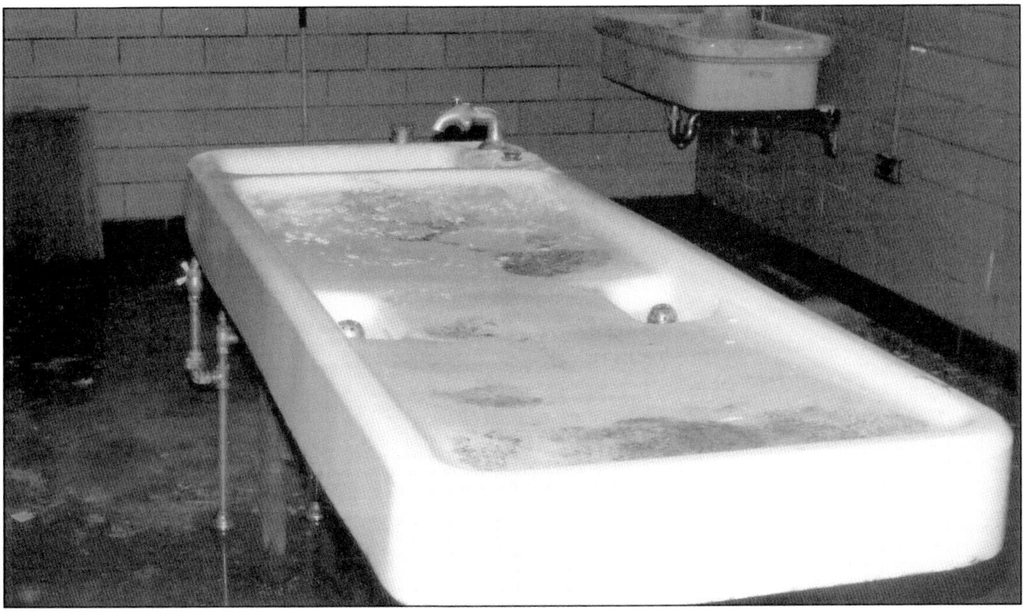

One of the biggest reasons why the laboratory was broken into so often was because it was adjacent to the morgue. This mortuary table was one of the badges of courage for urban explorers to find and photograph. Note the puddles of water surrounding the base of the table. The ground level of the Hutchinson Building was extremely damp because of poor drainage. The basement was completely inaccessible because it was filled with stagnant water.

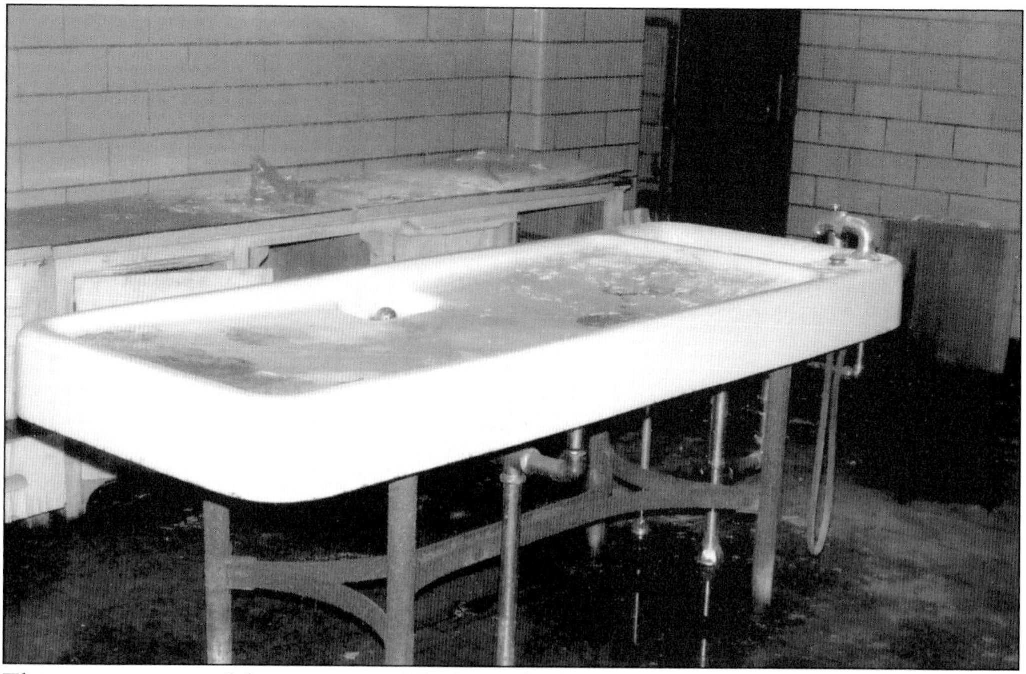

This opposite view of the mortuary table shows the drains and sink system. In September 2002, the table and four-unit morgue freezer were sold at an online auction for about $500. The table was reportedly sold to create a bar in someone's home. Although patients did die at Dixmont, autopsies were relatively rare—one or two reported each year, usually related to suicides. Many patients simply died of heart disease and other natural causes.

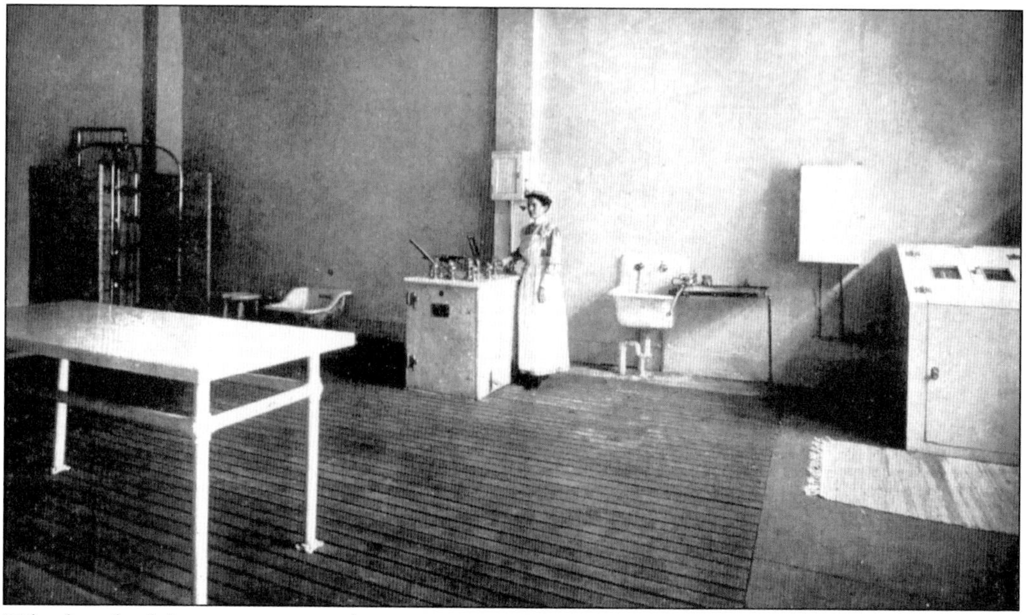

Whether the laboratory was modern or vintage, Dixmont was always prepared to treat patients with the leading methods of the times. This photograph shows the hydrotherapy department at Dixmont. Hydrotherapy was a popular means of treating delirium tremens in the 1930s. The regime included complete withdrawal from alcohol, cold sheet packs, and a high calorie diet.

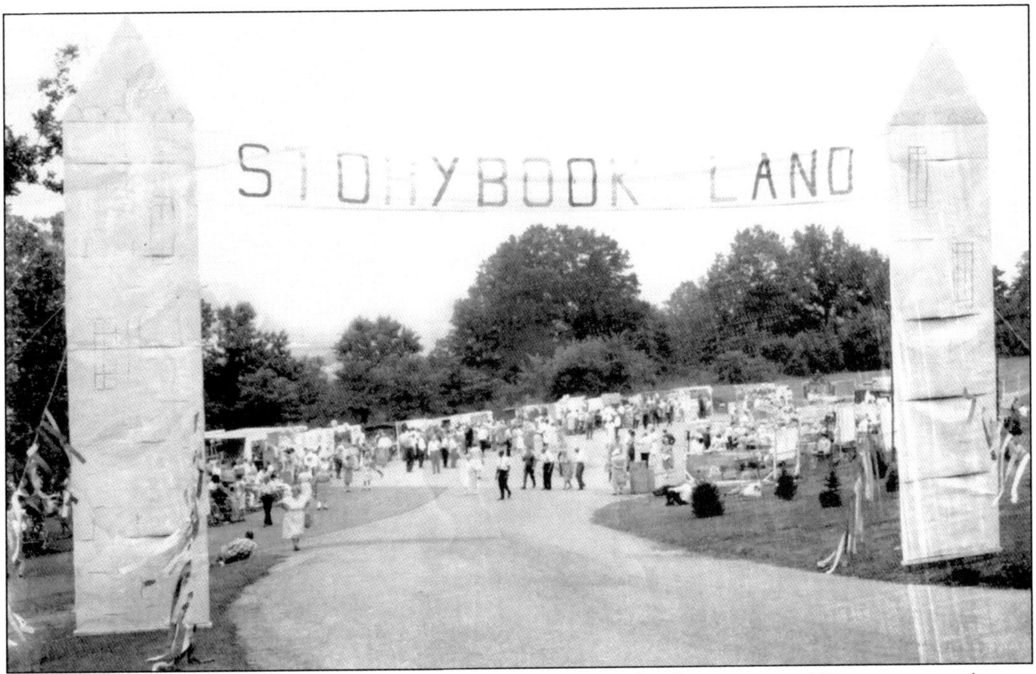

This photograph shows one of the great carnivals put on for the patients. Themes were chosen from a variety of sources, but, according to volunteer coordinator Helen Wolf, generally followed a Disneyland motif. Staff and volunteers created elaborate sets for these festivals, such as the gates of Storybook Land shown here. (Courtesy Helen Wolf.)

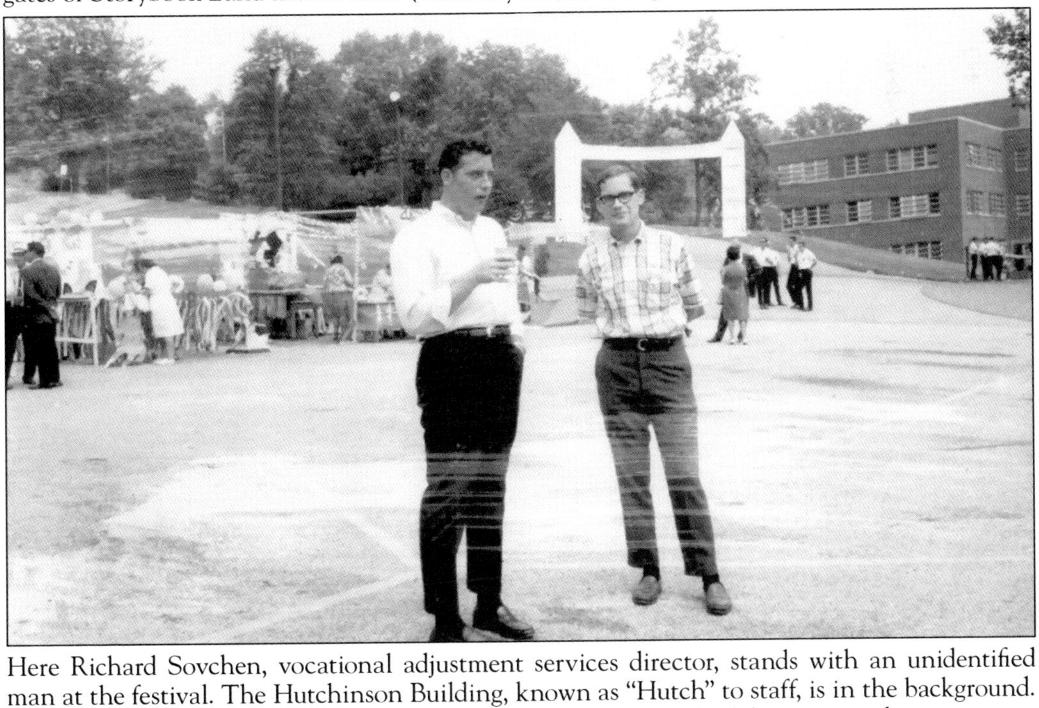

Here Richard Sovchen, vocational adjustment services director, stands with an unidentified man at the festival. The Hutchinson Building, known as "Hutch" to staff, is in the background. The first floor windows behind the sloping hillside are where the laboratory and morgue were located. (Courtesy Helen Wolf.)

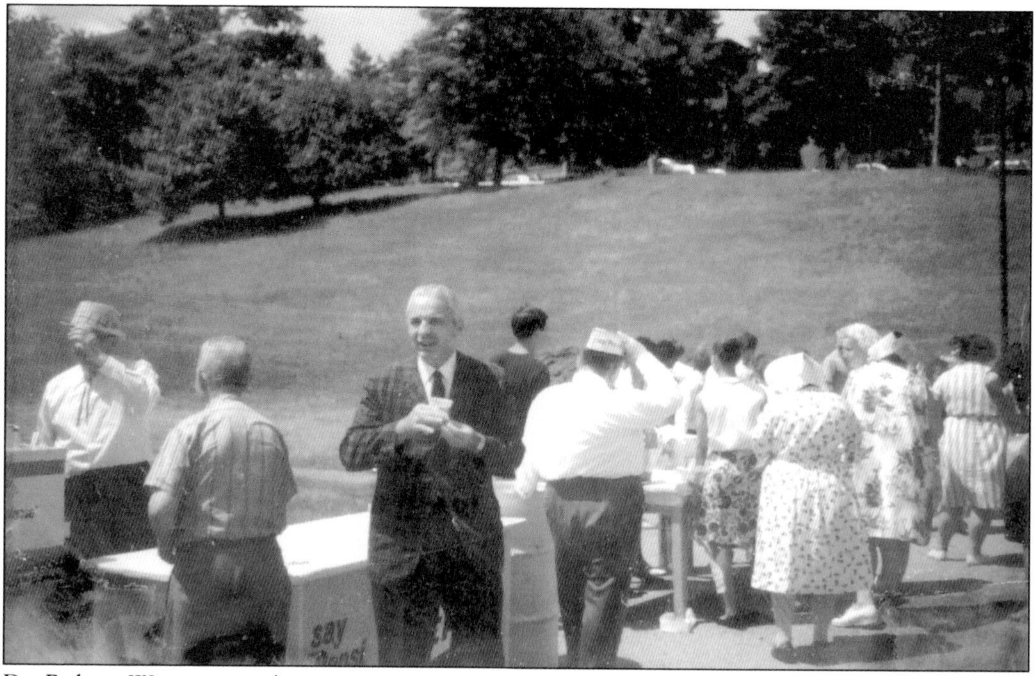

Dr. Robert Weimer stands among patients and volunteers during one of Dixmont's carnivals. The carnivals were annual events, typically held in July, and volunteers usually provided more than 1,000 hours of service to carry out the events. (Courtesy Helen Wolf.)

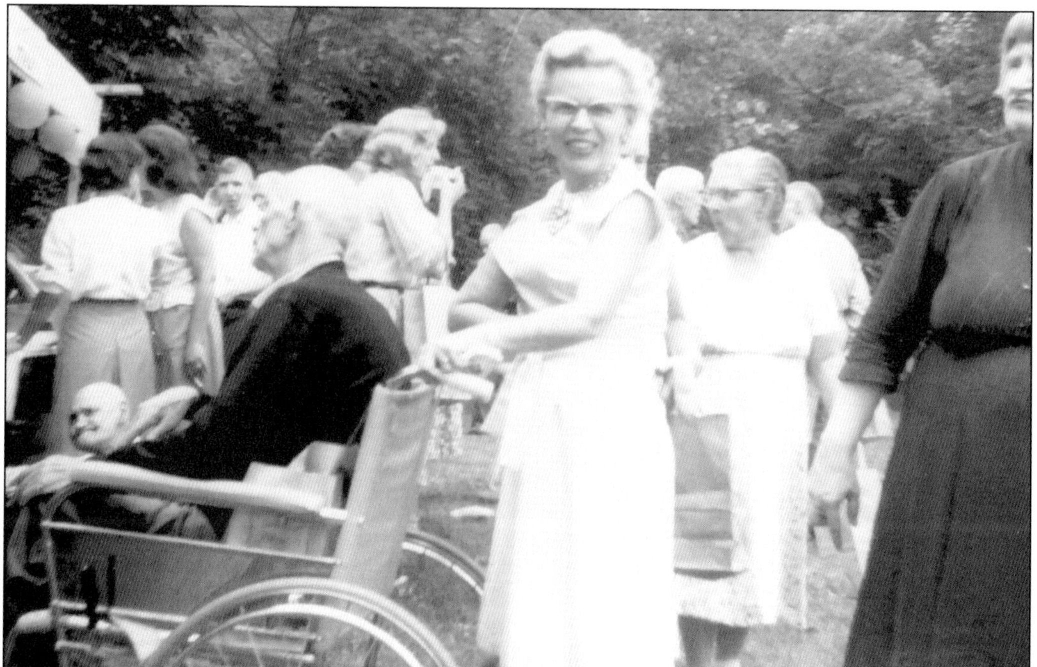

Often volunteers became employees at Dixmont. Here Florence Bayan, a long-term volunteer at Dixmont, pushes an elderly patient from carnival booth to carnival booth. She later became a telephone operator in the administration department. (Courtesy Helen Wolf.)

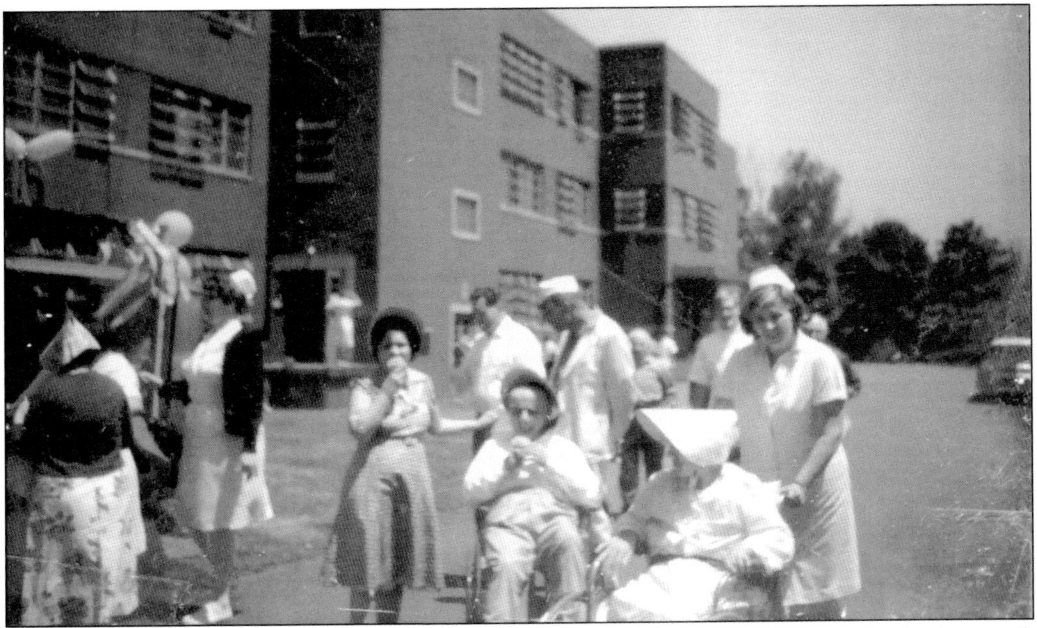

This photograph of patients and nurses shows a vibrant Hutchinson Building in the background. Because of its location, the Hutchinson Building could have been subject to creative reuse much like the Cammarata Building. However, age and neglect ruined the building to the point where renovation would have been too costly to consider. By the time the property was put up for sale by the state, the building was assessed to be worthless. (Courtesy Helen Wolf.)

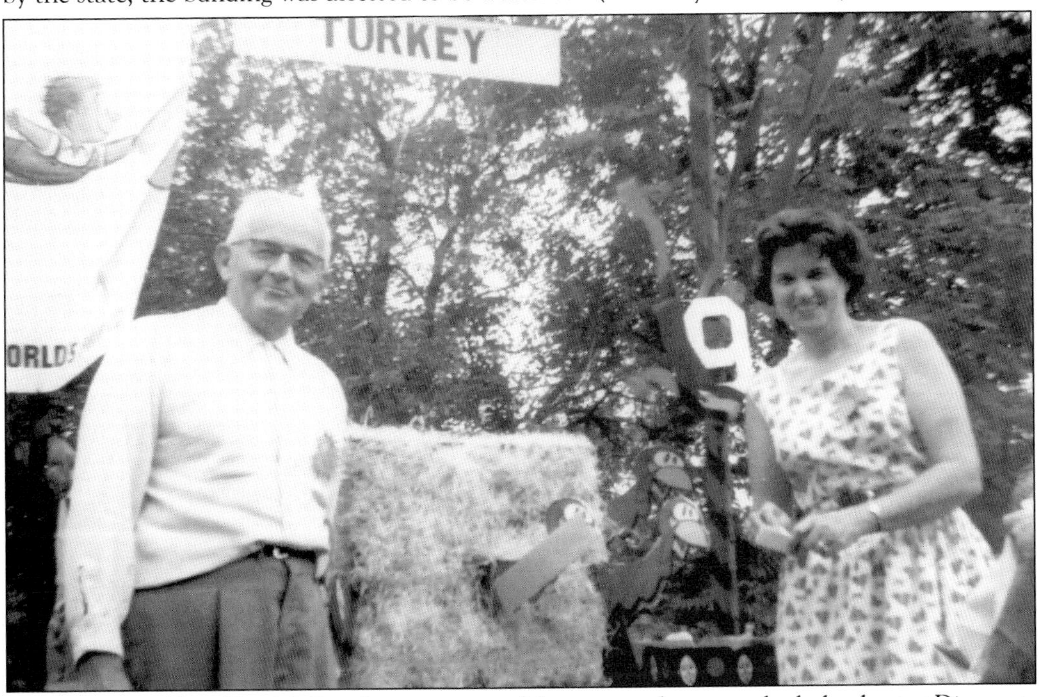

Robert Fitzgerald and Pat McGaughey were two of the many volunteers who helped out at Dixmont. The "small world" theme of this carnival is obvious from the Turkey tag on the booth. Other carnival themes included the Roaring Twenties and Storybook Land. (Courtesy Helen Wolf.)

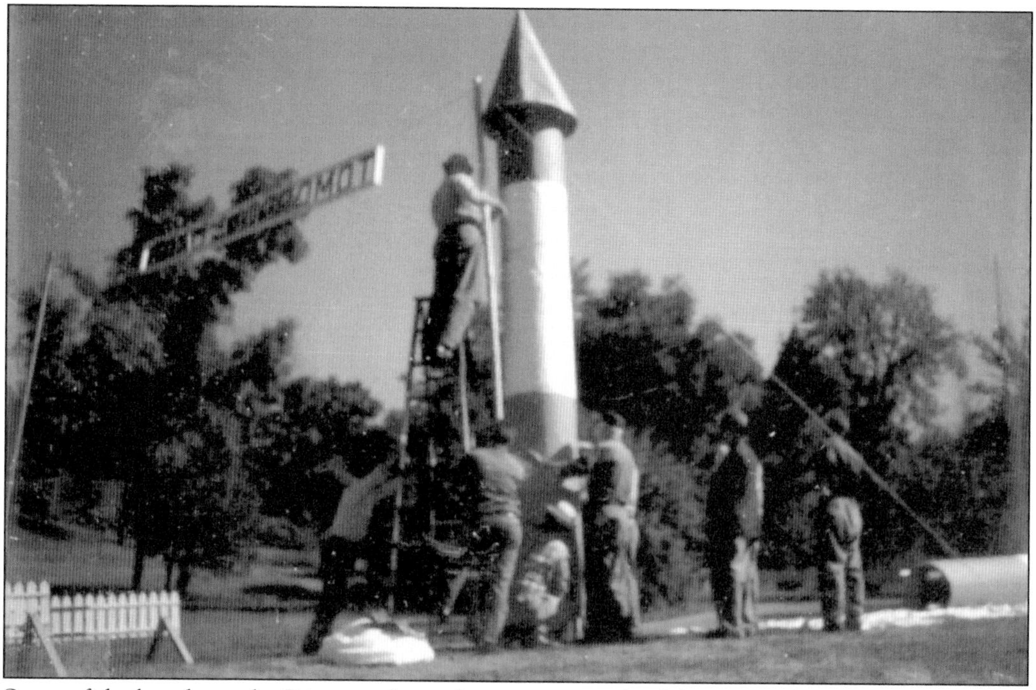

Some of the booths at the Dixmont festivals were extremely elaborate and complicated to build. Here volunteers erect a large rocket for display. This particular carnival was held in July 1966. (Courtesy Helen Wolf.)

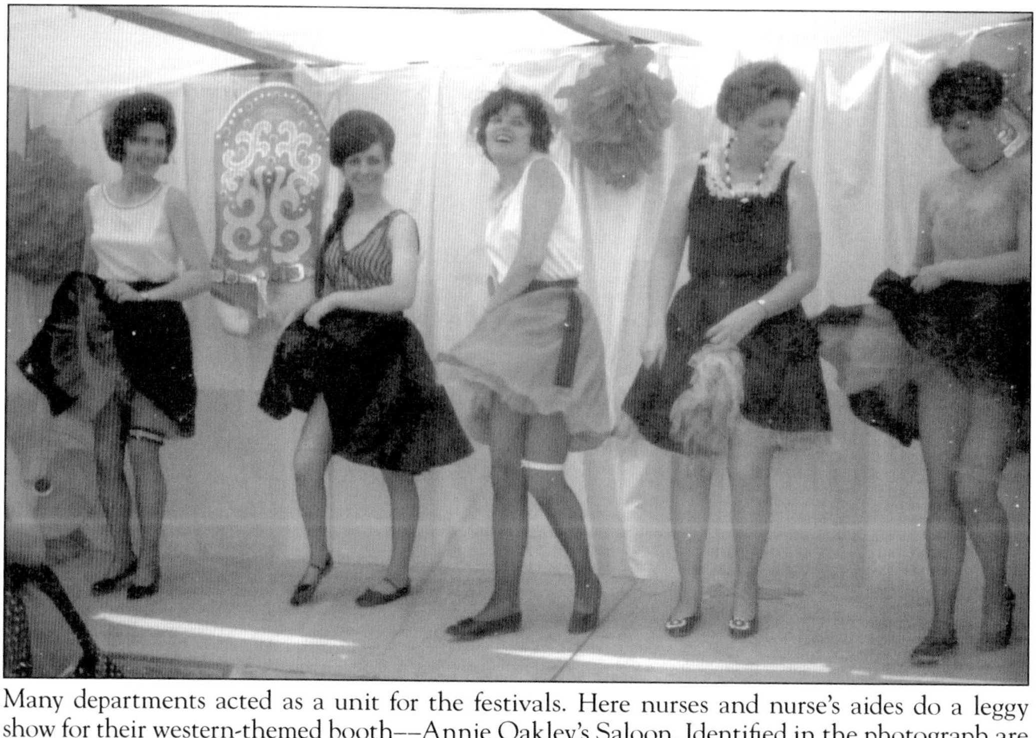

Many departments acted as a unit for the festivals. Here nurses and nurse's aides do a leggy show for their western-themed booth––Annie Oakley's Saloon. Identified in the photograph are Dorothy Swinotek, far left, and G. Klemantovich, far right. (Courtesy Helen Wolf.)

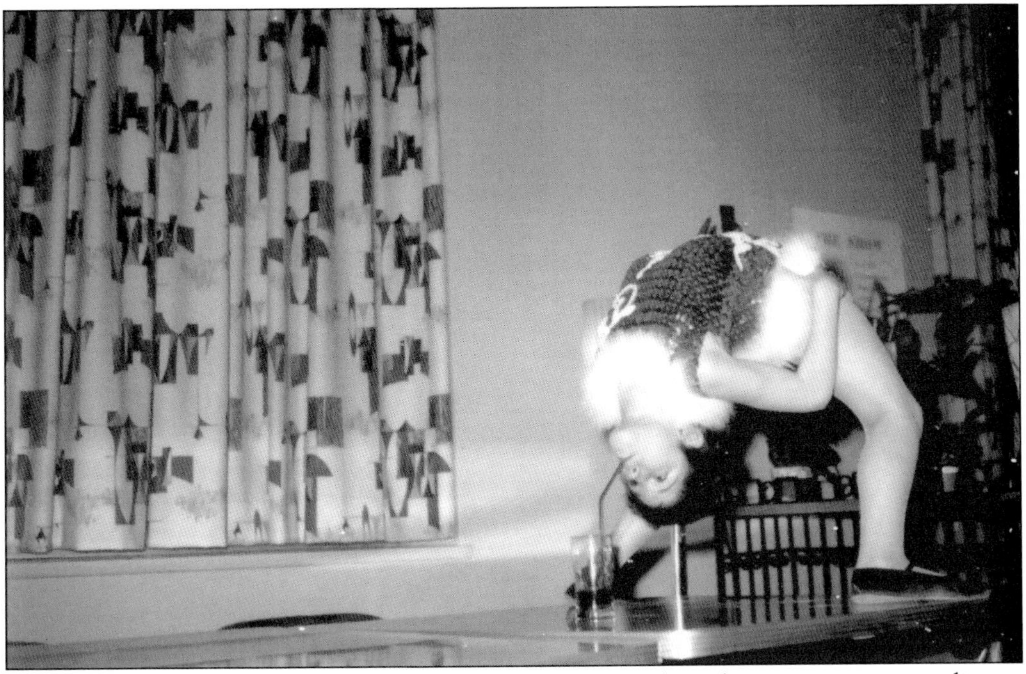

This unidentified volunteer performs an elaborate stunt at the volunteer appreciation dinner. Volunteers were key to Dixmont's survival. More than 120 participated in the recreation program and more than 60 volunteered with nursing service. (Courtesy Helen Wolf.)

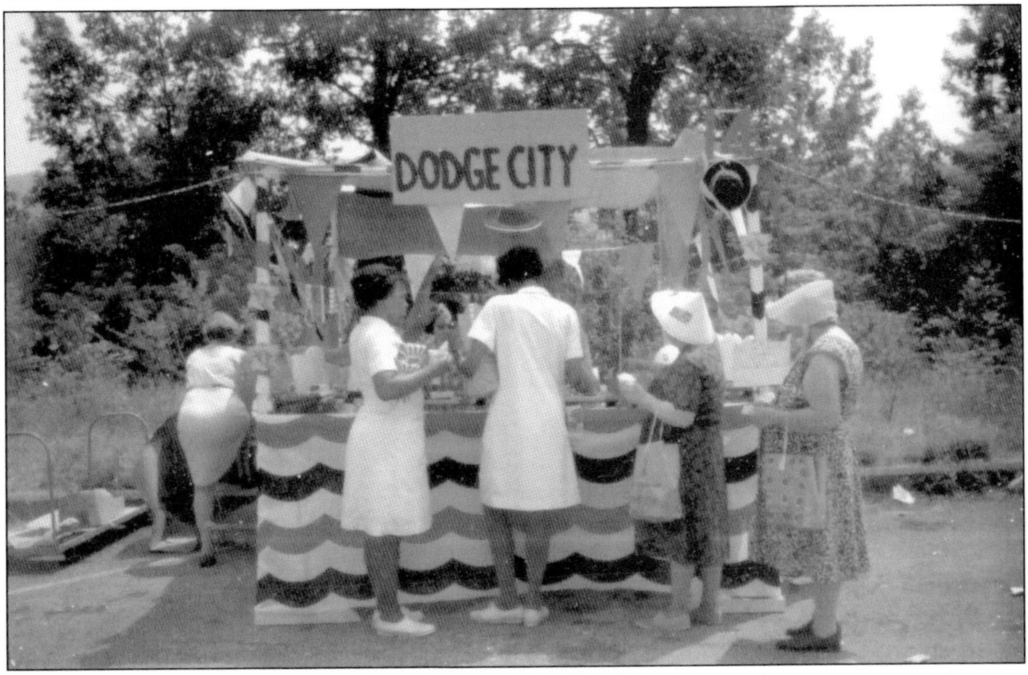

Community groups such as the Sewickley YMCA offered services, such as reserving swimming pool time. The Sewickley Valley and Beaver County Mental Health Associations helped out with Dixmont's mission by offering support services. Here patients line up at a booth during the carnival, which was put on by volunteer efforts. (Courtesy Helen Wolf.)

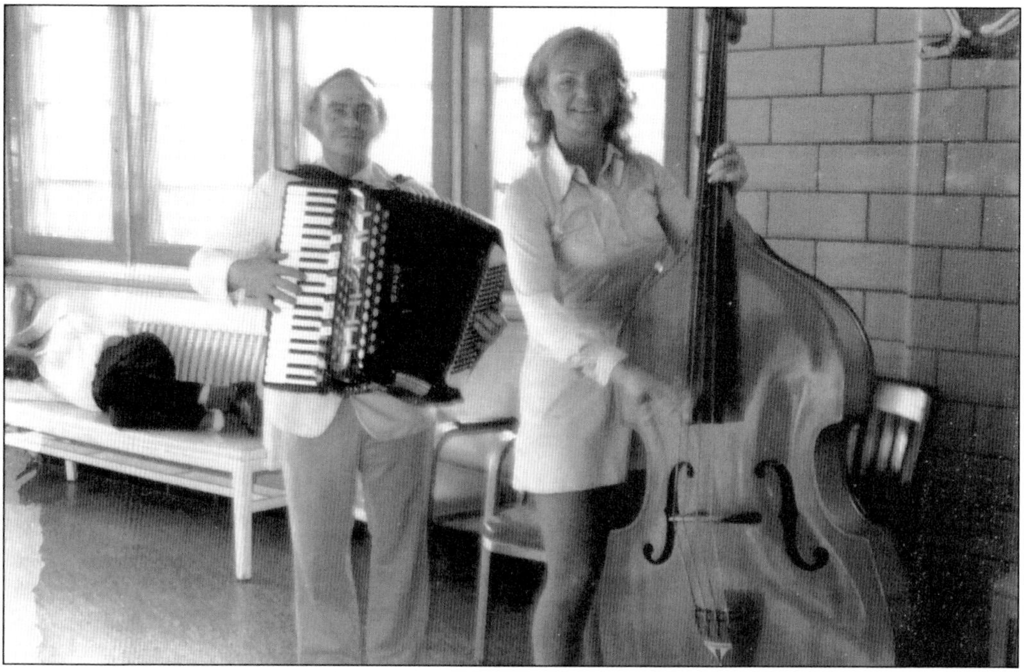

These two volunteers, the Aiellos, were enthusiastic musicians who visited Dixmont monthly to perform music in the Hutchinson Building. Other musical acts to visit Dixmont included the Chet Sporney Band. On occasion, patients would receive tickets to outside concerts, such as Ella Fitzgerald or performances of *My Fair Lady*. (Courtesy Helen Wolf.)

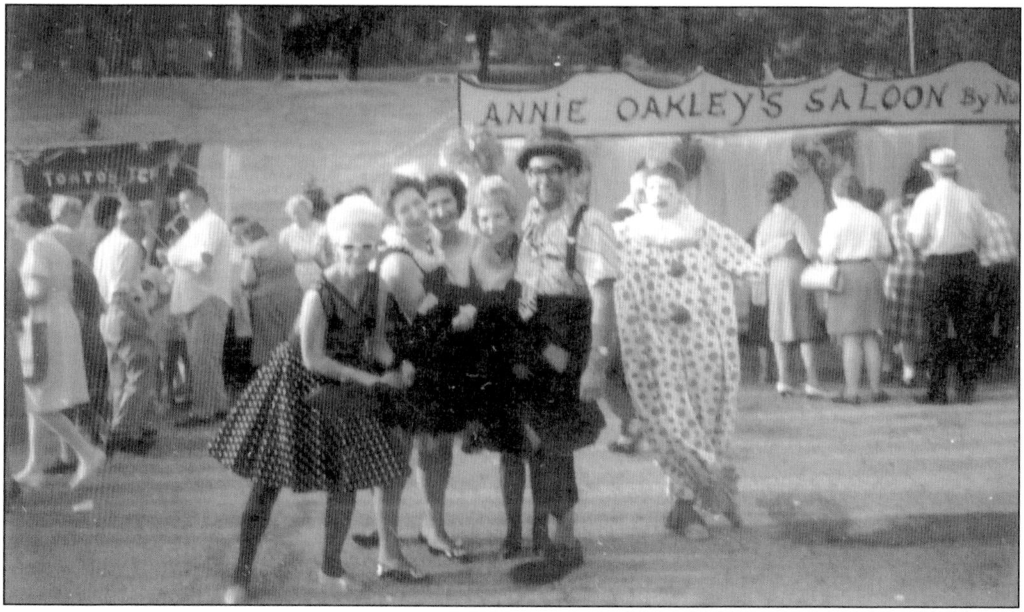

In addition to staff and volunteers, community groups were always willing to help out the patients of Dixmont. Many clowns were Shriners, who would come to entertain. Despite Dixmont's tranquil isolation, it was never far from the communities it served. Knights of Columbus, Salvation Army, Missionary Circle, and other volunteer groups all donated to Dixmont's cause. (Courtesy Helen Wolf.)

Three

The Art of Healing

Art is a natural function of the human mind, whether it is the fractal-based abstractions of Jackson Pollock or the visual riddles of René Magritte. The universality of art was not lost on the staff and patients of Dixmont. Having a large deaf unit, founded on July 24, 1972, many Dixmont patients lived in a world of vision only. The art in Dixmont was conceived across all mediums, from crafts and handwork to murals and displays of celebration. Much of this work was evaluated by the Therapeutic Environment Committee, which sought to rehabilitate patients through relaxed surroundings. The committee was first called to order at 1:30 p.m. on June 27, 1979, by chairman C. W. Daugherty. The committee was unique in that it sought out and involved patient input through patient representatives.

After Dixmont closed, the site became the site of another kind of expression—that of graffiti. Ralph Stroyne endeavored, through the help of local artists, to create one last, large-scale installation that would stand the test of time.

Weaving beneath the Dixmont property was a cement tunnel. Plans for the shopping center on the site called for sealing a part of the tunnel instead of demolishing it. Stroyne put advertisements on the Internet calling for an entry fee to any artist willing to create a work on the walls of the tunnel to create an artistic "time capsule."

The project got publicity, but no acclaim. The majority of artists were simply local people wanting a pass to spray paint an old asylum. Some drove in from other states and worked overnight to complete their designs. In the end, the tunnel was sealed.

However, much of the real art of Dixmont endured. Murals from the 1940s were unveiled as modern paint peeled back from exposure. It was almost as if there were layers of artistic sediment buried by coats of paint. From the days of Dr. Joseph Allison Reed to Dixmont's Renaissance under Dr. Robert Weimer, art was always an integral part of patient rehabilitation.

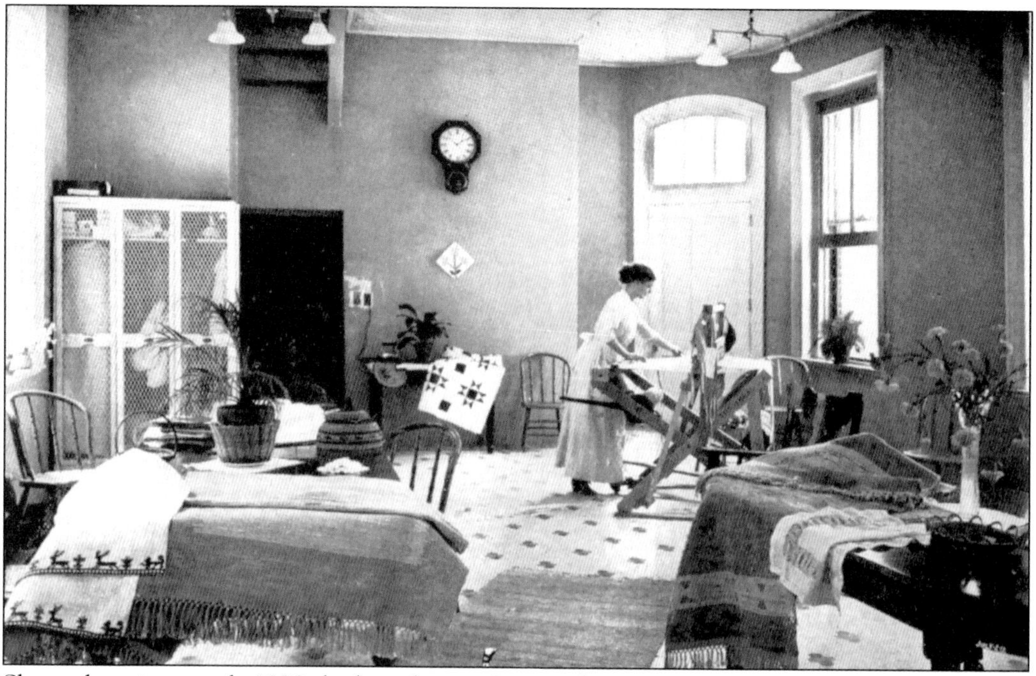

Shown here is an early 1900s look at the art therapy department at Dixmont. The department, in the early 1900s, mainly practiced fabric arts: knitting, quilting, rug making, weaving, crocheting, embroidering, cross-stitching, and tatting. The department also produced appliqué, baskets, lamp shades, and flower items such as boutonnieres.

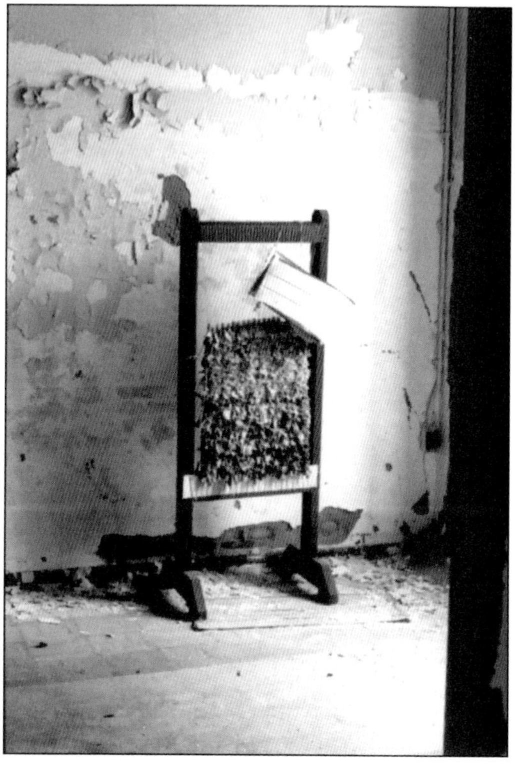

This loom and rag rug stood long after Dixmont was closed. Even in its early years, Dixmont's occupational therapy was extremely productive. During the Civil War, 100 shirts were made for the troops fighting for the North. During times of peace, everything from doilies and rugs to quilts and baby cloths were fashioned by patient hands.

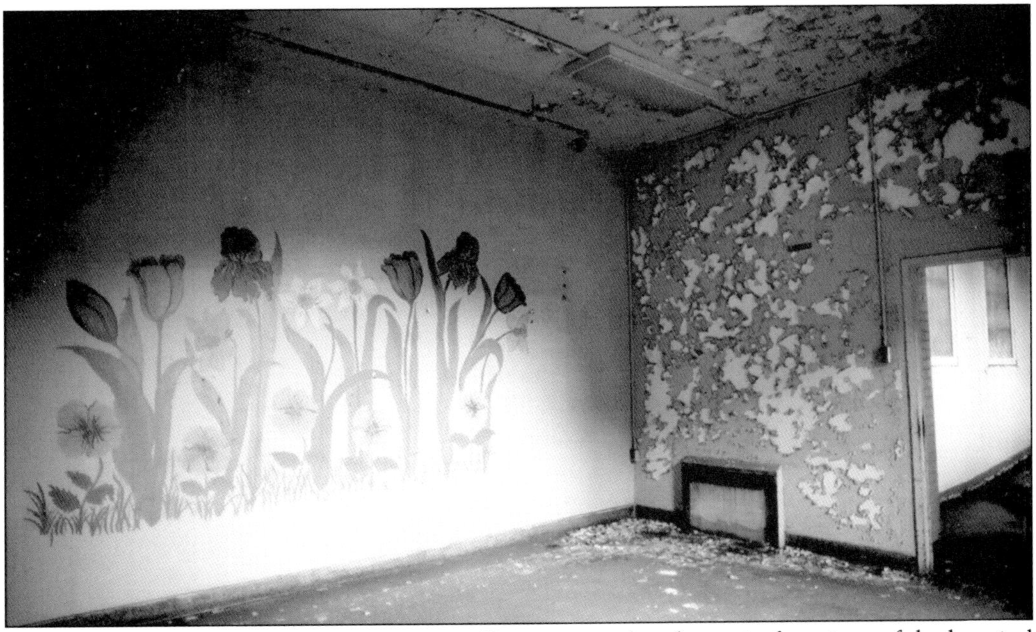

The therapeutic environment committee at Dixmont analyzed certain functions of the hospital and made recommendations to the superintendent. Some of those recommendations were wall murals, of which Dixmont had many. Some murals were painted over, only to be rediscovered in a closed hospital when the top layer of paint began to curl back. Here this flower mural was painted in Reed Hall near one of the ramps to the dietary building.

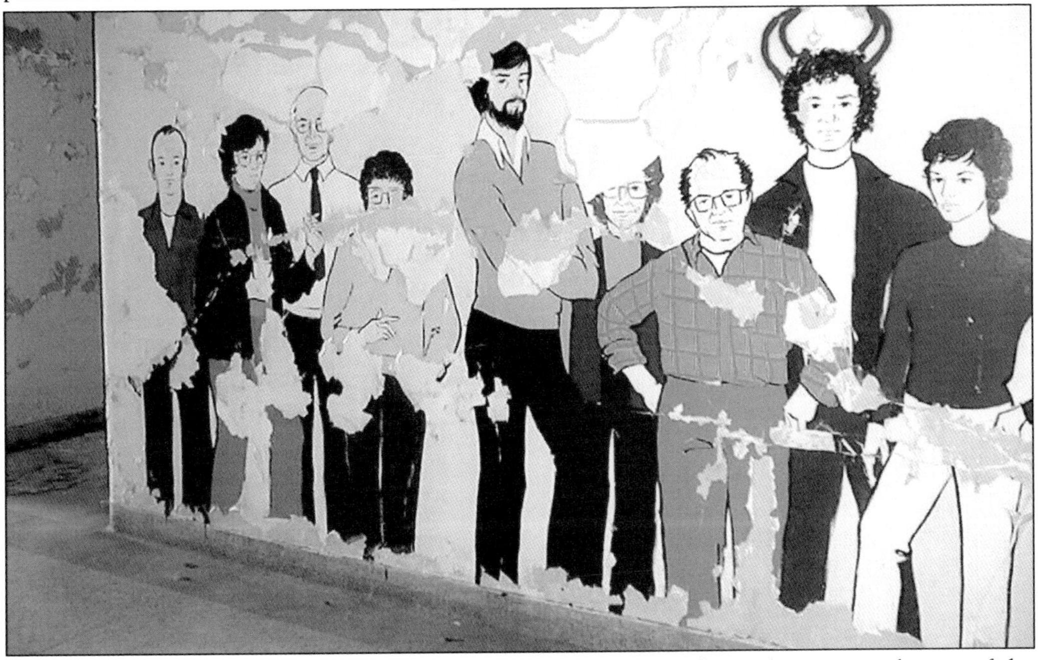

While many murals were defaced over time, some still portray the enthusiasm and spirit of the employees who worked at Dixmont. This mural is of employees working at the hospital at the time. According to surviving employees, the sixth person from the left originally had a bird on top of her head because a patient suggested it might look nice.

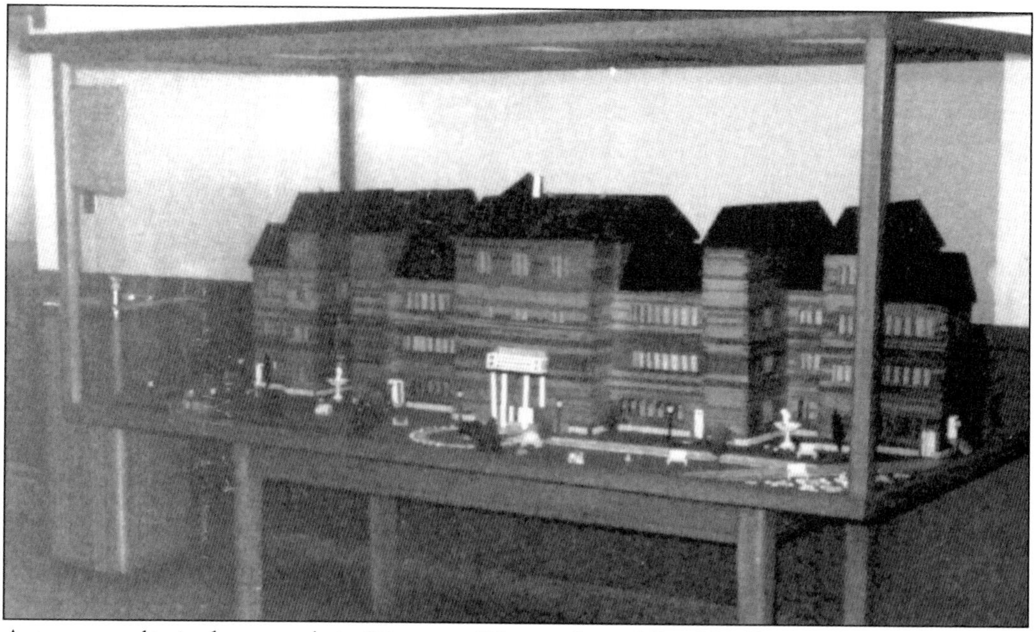

Art was not limited to murals in Dixmont. This replica of Reed Hall is made from wood and stood under glass inside the real Reed Hall. The replica was created by an employee of the hospital. The occupational therapy department used household items such as egg crates, bleach bottles, and felt to help patients create their own works of art. Pleas for materials were regularly published in the volunteer newsletters. (Courtesy Tracy Ferguson.)

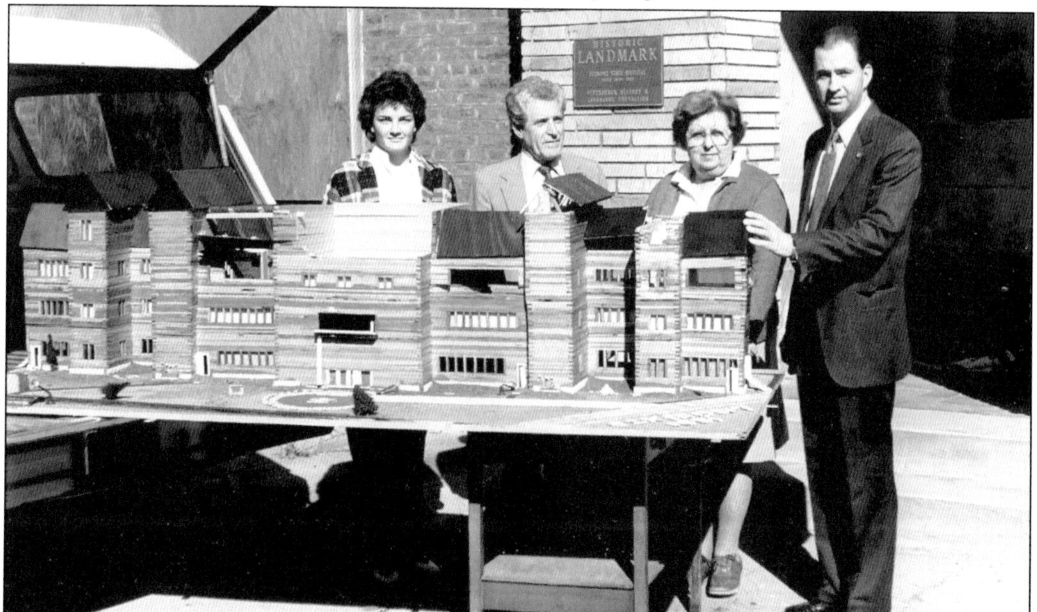

The Reed Hall replica was later donated to the Western Pennsylvania Hospital. Pictured here from left to right are Tracy Weimer, daughter of Dr. Robert Weimer; unidentified; Gladys Phillips, a historian for the Ben Avon Area Historical Association; and David J. Mayernik, former state representative. (Courtesy Connie Rankin/the Citizen; photograph by Earl Rankin.)

Dixmont's history of artwork lasted long after the hospital closed. As the years passed, layers of paint peeled from the walls, revealing past generations of murals. Here a mixed-media creation will last forever in an art time capsule within the tunnel system beneath Dixmont. Part of the tunnel was demolished in the commercial development of the site; however, one section was simply sealed. In 2002, the Stroyne family opened the property up to artists to partake in the time capsule.

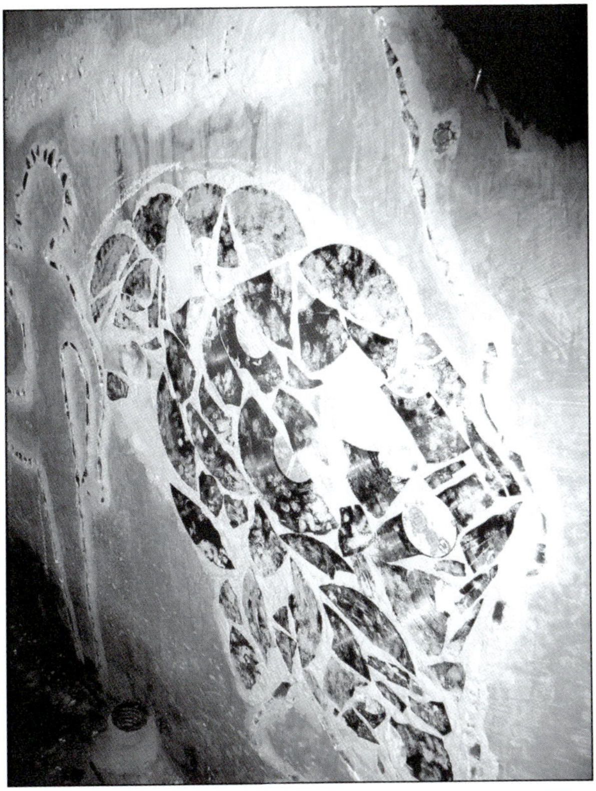

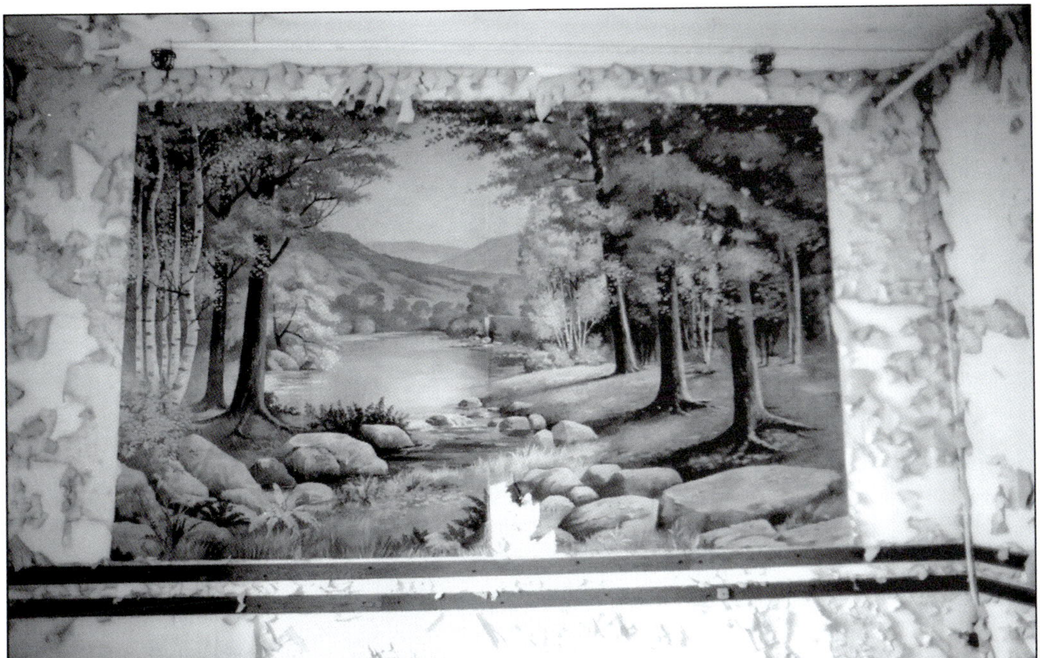

Not all murals were hand painted. Some, such as this one, which was on a wall on the first floor of Reed Hall, were commercially produced wallpaper products. This mural was later found to be defaced in subsequent trips to the site.

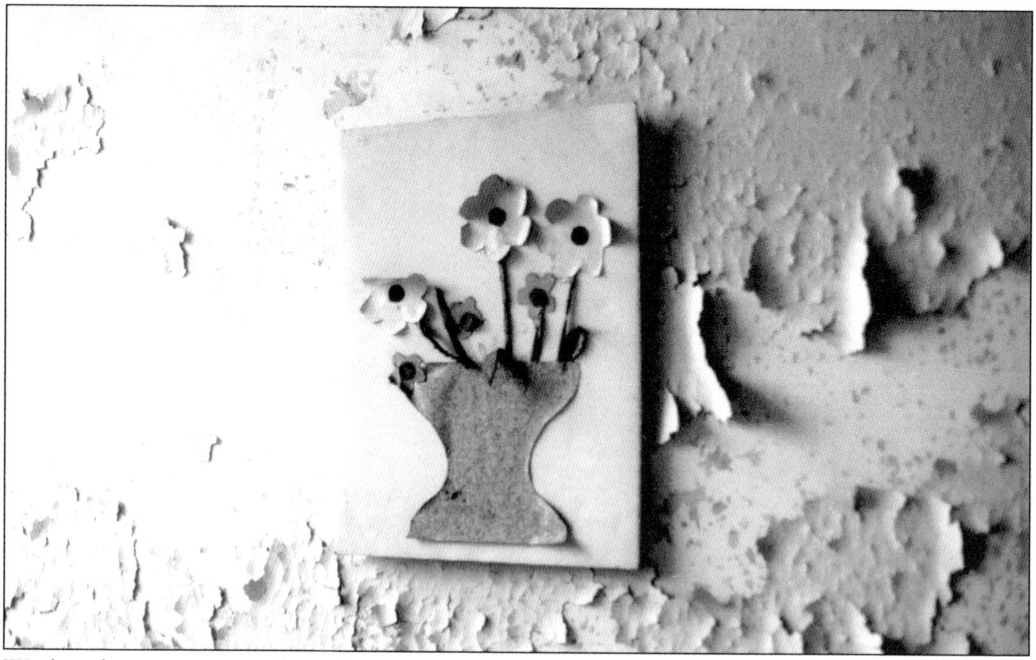

Works of patient art, such as this cut-paper flowers in a vase, were simply left in Dixmont's various rooms. While they have importance as to how art played a role in patient therapy, they also speak volumes to the swiftness with which Dixmont closed.

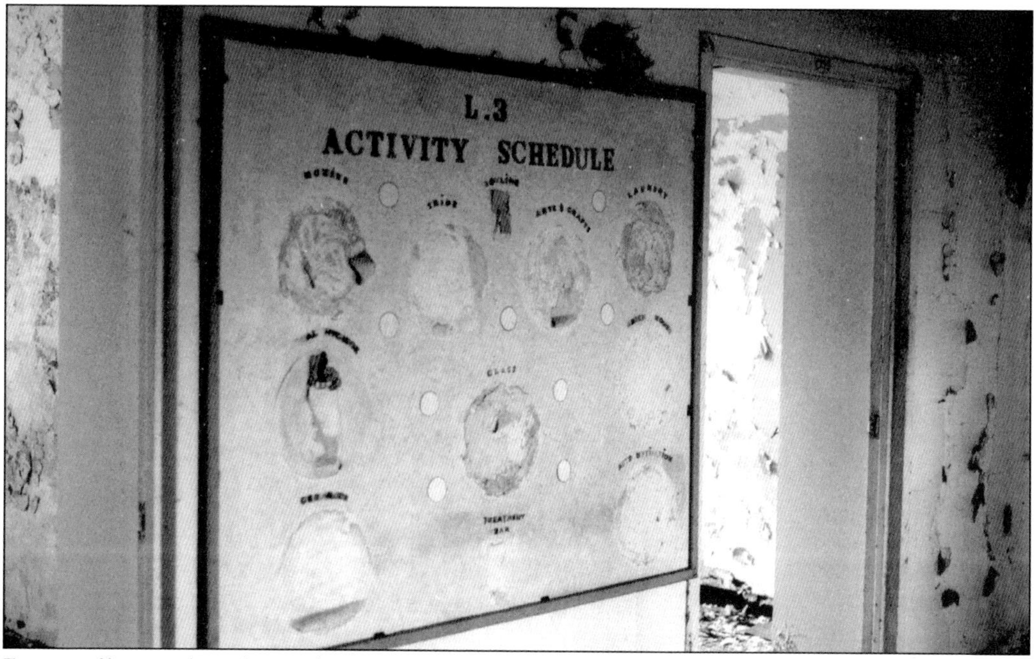

Even staff-created works, such as this Lawrence Unit 3 activities chart, were simply frozen in time when Tom Patton locked the doors of Reed Hall in 1984. Activities available to patients included punching heavy bags to reduce emotional stress, weekly swimming and bowling trips, and outdoor recreation that was comprised of 20 minutes each of exercise and active and passive games.

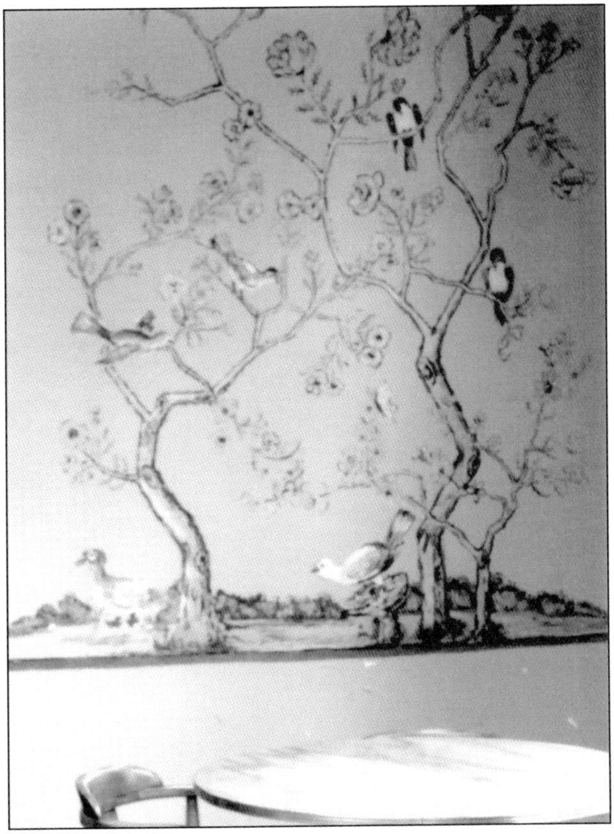

This mural was painted in the dietary building on a wall near the staff cafeteria. The creation of a staff cafeteria was a goal set by Dr. Robert Weimer in 1974. The dietary department took patient nourishment very seriously. Decaffeinated coffee was served to patients. Each patient had a nutritional assessment. Patients were placed on high fiber diets to reduce the reliance on laxatives. (Courtesy Tracy Ferguson.)

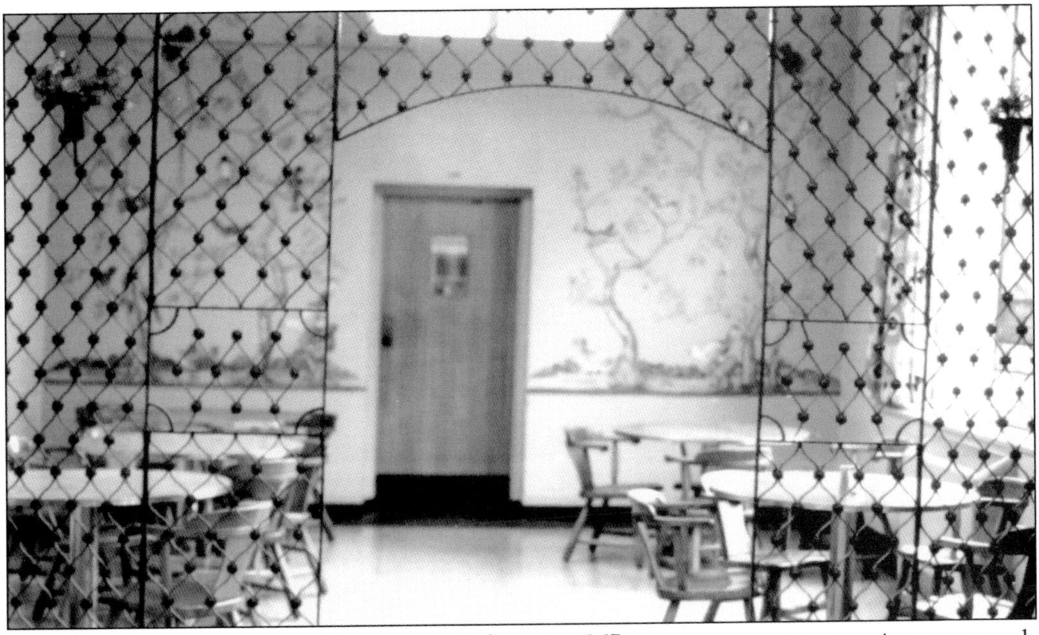

When the bars were removed from the windows in 1967, some were put to creative reuse, such as this room divider. Other bars were converted into planters. This room-dividing gate separates the cafeteria from the kitchen hallway in the dietary building. (Courtesy Tracy Ferguson.)

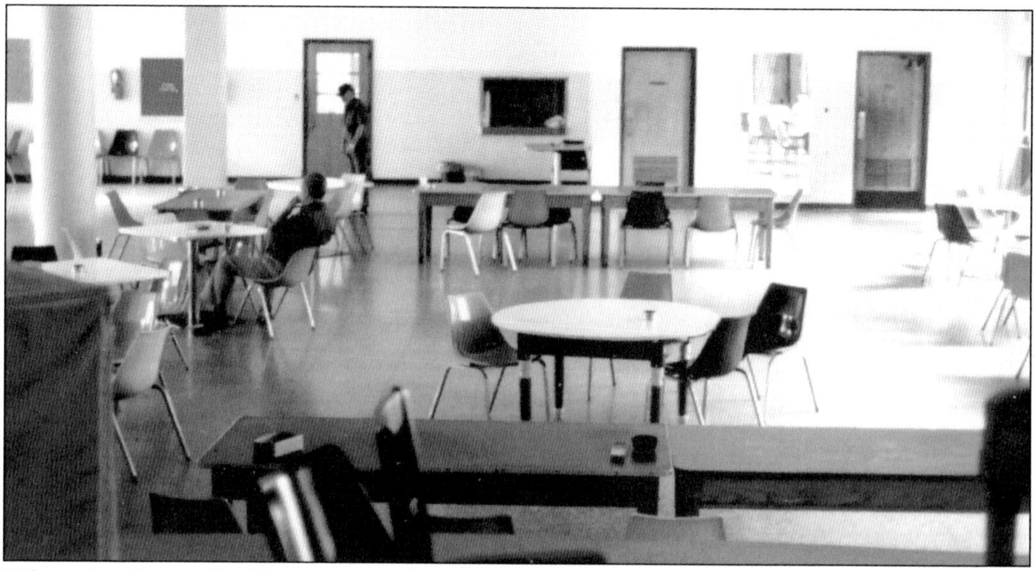

When the dietary building was not being used for recognition dinners, it was the everyday cafeteria for patients and staff. However, as with all large food preparation operations, the building did have its occasional problems with roaches. Records indicate that food carts were "bombed" after the evening meals and cleaned for use the next morning. At times, exterminators were coming every two weeks to spray.

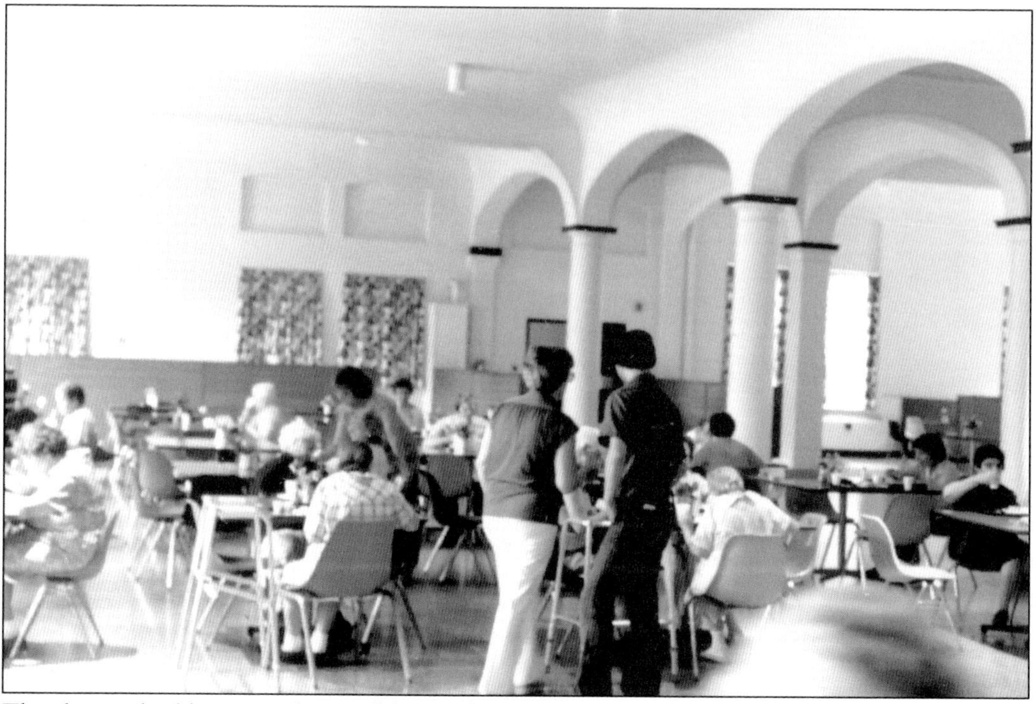

The dietary building was designed by Frederick John Osterling, famous in Pittsburgh for his architecture. The building was classic early 1900s institutional in design and was connected to Reed Hall by way of two elevated walkways. There is a third floor to the building that once served as staff quarters.

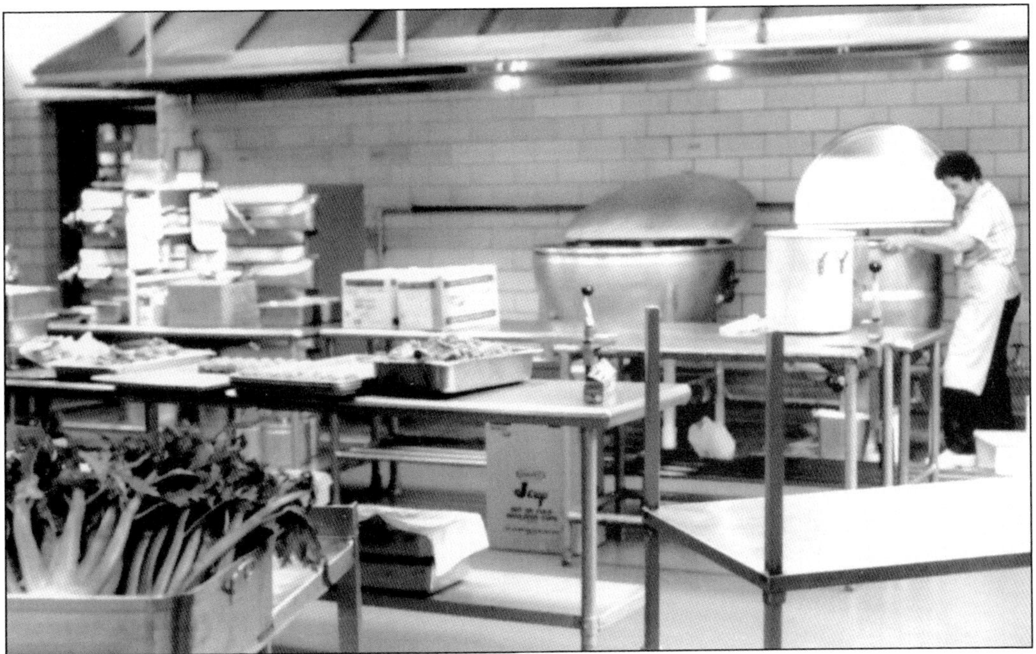

Between the two dining rooms was the kitchen. Shown here, the kitchen staff was charged with feeding hundreds of patients and staff daily to the tune of 11,000 meals per week. The kitchen also served as a transitional area for patients moving toward normal community living through the Vocational Adjustment Services program. (Courtesy Tracy Ferguson.)

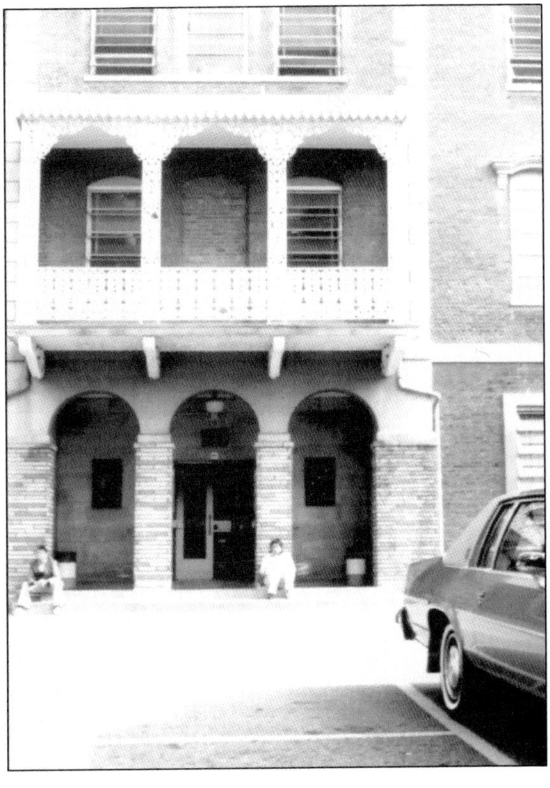

Reed Hall's cast-iron balcony was in itself a work of art. The balcony was salvaged and sold to an antiques collector in Chicago by the Stroyne Family Limited Partnership. Ralph Stroyne said he actually sold the balcony twice––once to an antiques collector in Zelienople who never came to pick it up. The collector from Chicago paid around $2,000 for the piece, Stroyne said.

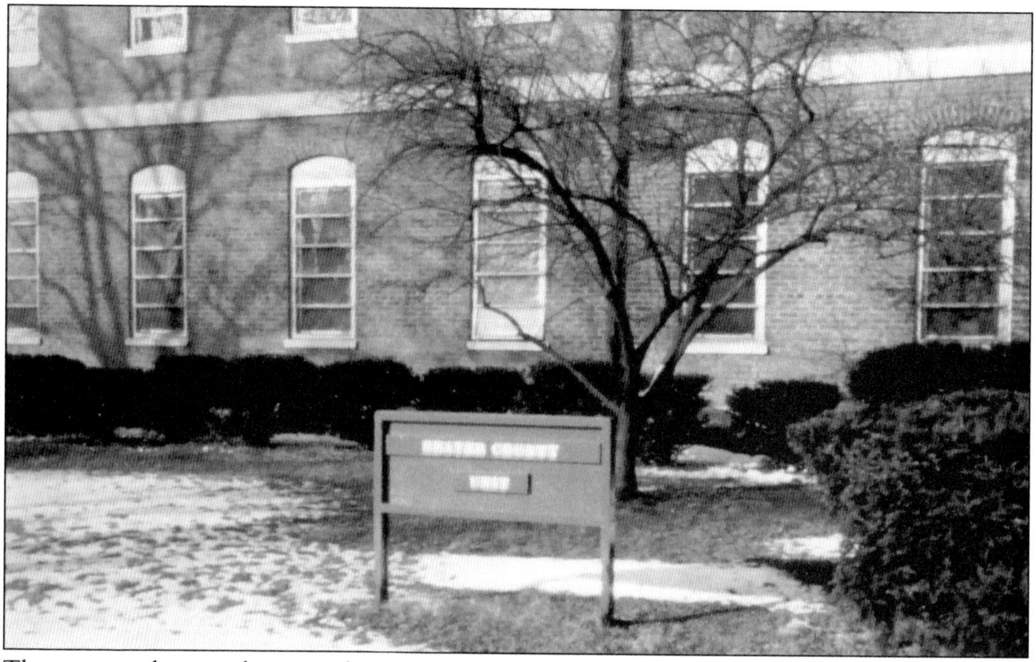

This picture shows a directional sign outside of Reed Hall. Dr. Robert Weimer endeavored to improve the grounds despite budget cuts. The roads at Dixmont were given formal names under Weimer's tenure, and in 1971, more than 60 streetlights were installed throughout the campus. (Courtesy Tracy Ferguson.)

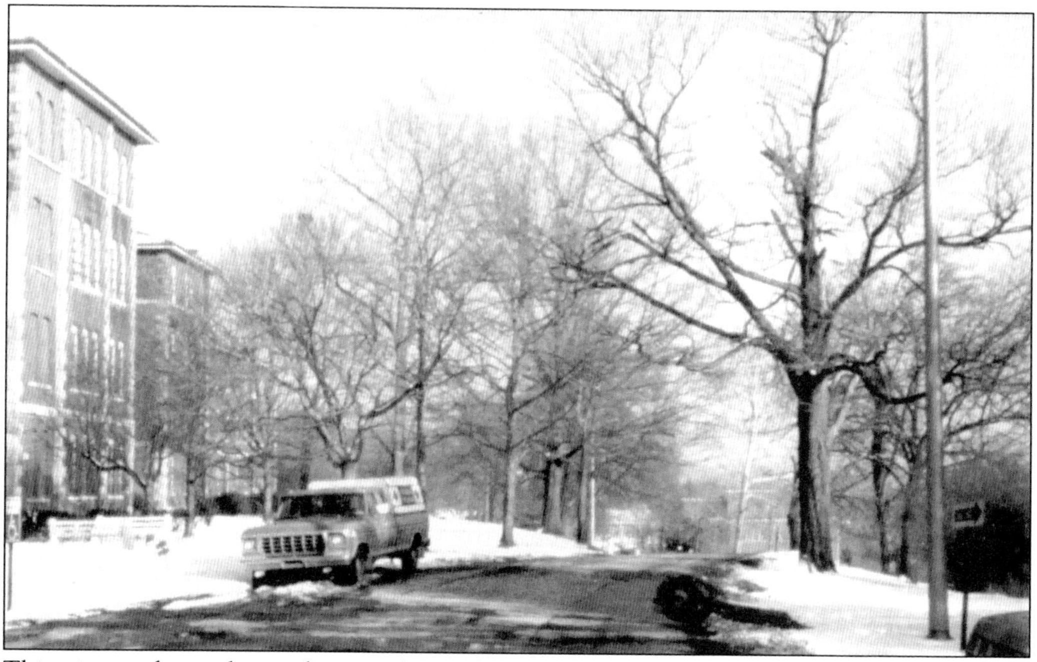

This picture shows the roadway in front of Reed Hall. The focus on art and recreation was not based entirely within the Dixmont campus. Dixmont had a bus that circulated as many as three times each day to take patients to off-campus locations for resocialization. Such excursions included Sunday afternoon concerts to the Pittsburgh Symphony. (Courtesy Tracy Ferguson.)

Invitations went out from the Dixmont Board of Trustees for the April 30, 1954, groundbreaking of the admission and treatment building, later known as the Hutchinson Building. The board included Frank W. Ittel, president; Donald O. Bair Sr., vice president; Victor L. Alski; Robert G. Harris; Robert W. McDermott; Joseph F. Novak; Mary D. Phillips; James A. Robertson; and Eugene L. Youngue.

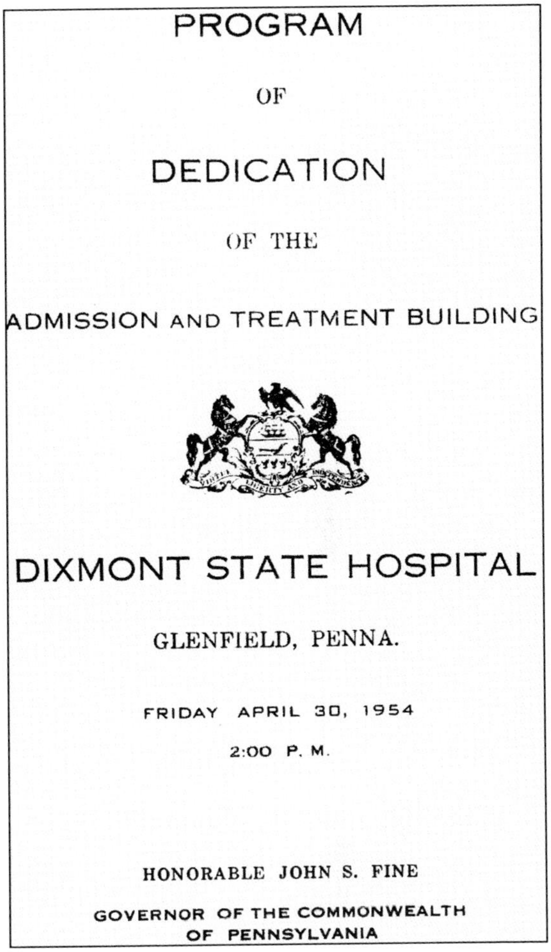

PROGRAM

OF

DEDICATION

OF THE

ADMISSION AND TREATMENT BUILDING

DIXMONT STATE HOSPITAL

GLENFIELD, PENNA.

FRIDAY APRIL 30, 1954

2:00 P. M.

HONORABLE JOHN S. FINE

GOVERNOR OF THE COMMONWEALTH OF PENNSYLVANIA

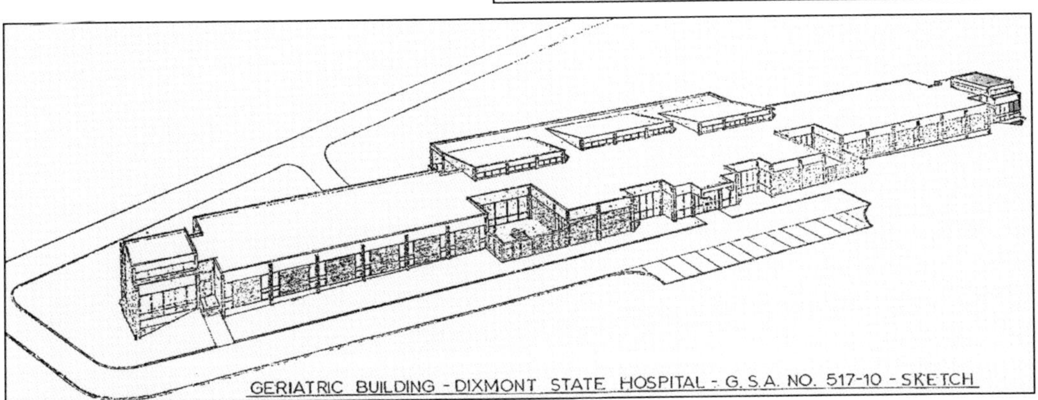

This drawing was the concept for the geriatric building at Dixmont. Intended to be the home to the hospital's aging population, the building later became known as the Cammarata Building, after Dr. Joseph Cammarata, predecessor to Dr. Robert Weimer as superintendent. Designed by William York Cocken and Cammarata himself, the building housed the volunteer department at various points of its existence and was situated in the neighboring borough of Emsworth (although still on a contiguous piece of Dixmont's property). This building is the only remaining structure left of Dixmont and is currently owned by the Stroyne family.

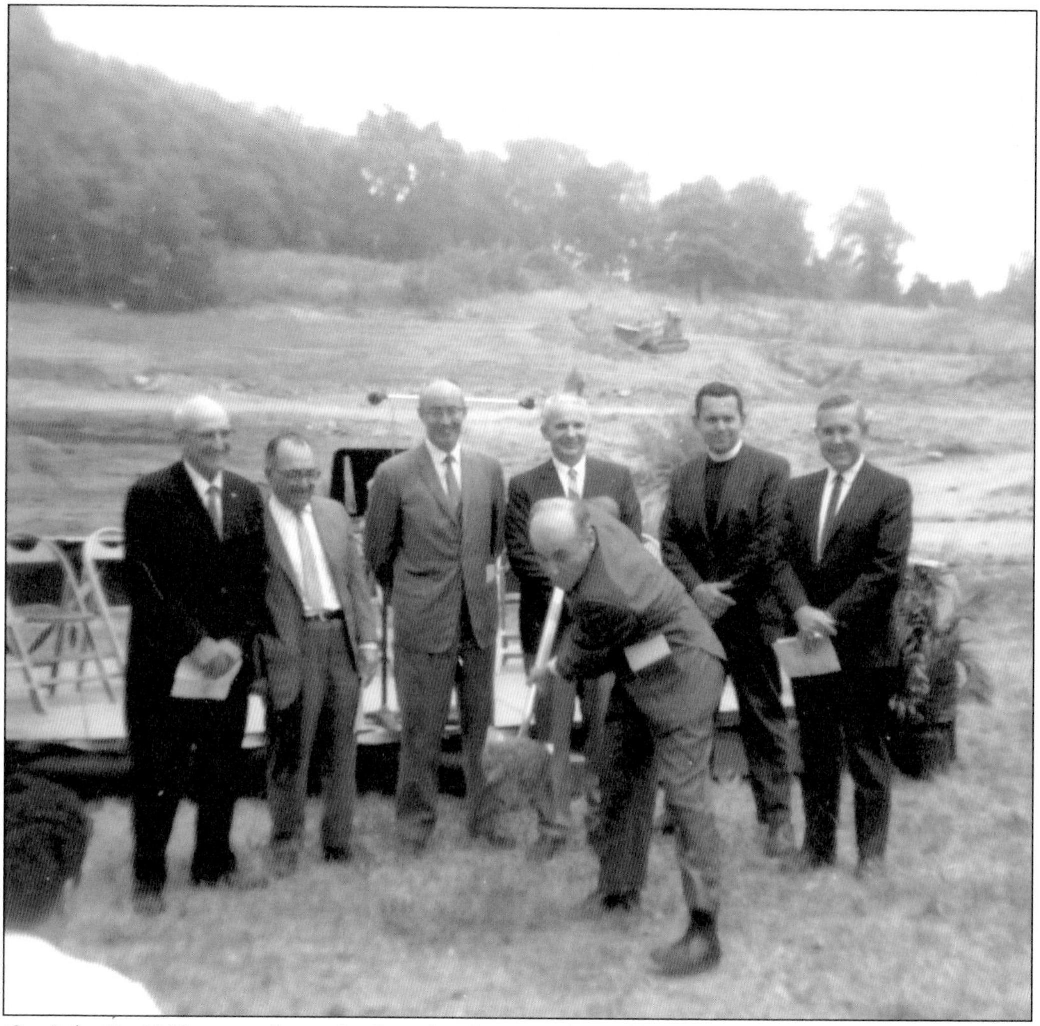

On July 11, 1969, ground was broken for the new $2 million geriatrics building at Dixmont. Pictured from left to right are Richard Shoup from the board of trustees, Dr. Joseph Cammarata, Dr. Charles C. Goodman, Dr. Robert Weimer, Pastor Charles Rampp, and Robert E. Lenker. Pennsylvania's deputy secretary of mental health, Joseph Adelstein, holds the shovel.

Four

DISINTEGRATION

It was not difficult to see that the Commonwealth of Pennsylvania was blatantly looking to shut down Dixmont, if not the entire Pennsylvania mental hospital network from 1950 on. Frustrated letters left the desk of superintendent Joseph Cammarata in the early 1960s asking for funding and simple fixes, such as asphalt for Dixmont's roads when the Pennsylvania Department of Transportation was working yards away on a Route 65 upgrade. These correspondences were denied outright. However, the state was willing to continue performing energy and utility reviews of Dixmont, which demonstrated how costly the hospital was because of its high ceilings and energy inefficient design.

In 1972, the state had come out and stated that Dixmont was to be shut down. Public outcry, however, led to a review of the plan, and Dixmont was granted a stay of execution. While the hospital was saved for the time being, subsequent years resulted in less and less money being allocated to Dixmont. This once vibrant and trailblazing hospital was being strangled shut by the state wallet chain.

By the time Dixmont closed in 1984, only a handful of its more than 80 structures were extant. The top two floors of Reed Hall were shut off from patient and staff use. Indeed, patient population declined as well. From more than 1,200 patients on the books at the end of 1940, to 745 at the end of 1967, to just 362 at the end of 1977, Dixmont was slowly growing vacant. The doors shut with 177 patients having to be transferred to Woodville and Mayview State Hospitals.

Despite the bleak outlook, correspondence from the superintendent and staff published in staff newsletters remained upbeat. Perhaps they grew accustomed to living under the shadow of a dying institution for so many years, or perhaps it was denial. Minutes of the Quality Assurance Committee of February 24, 1982, confirmed that rumors of Dixmont closing were still looming. The rumors were dispelled by Dr. Ezer H. Davis, who stated on record that there would simply be a consolidation of Woodville, Dixmont, and Mayview. Either way, the public support that bought hospitals such as Woodville a few extra years could not buy Dixmont any more time. In the June 1984 issue of *Sewickley Magazine*, Dr. Leroy Egan wrote that Dixmont had become "a symbol properly belonging to a different era." The hospital locked its doors for the last time on June 30, 1984, less than four months after a Valentine's Day announcement of its closing.

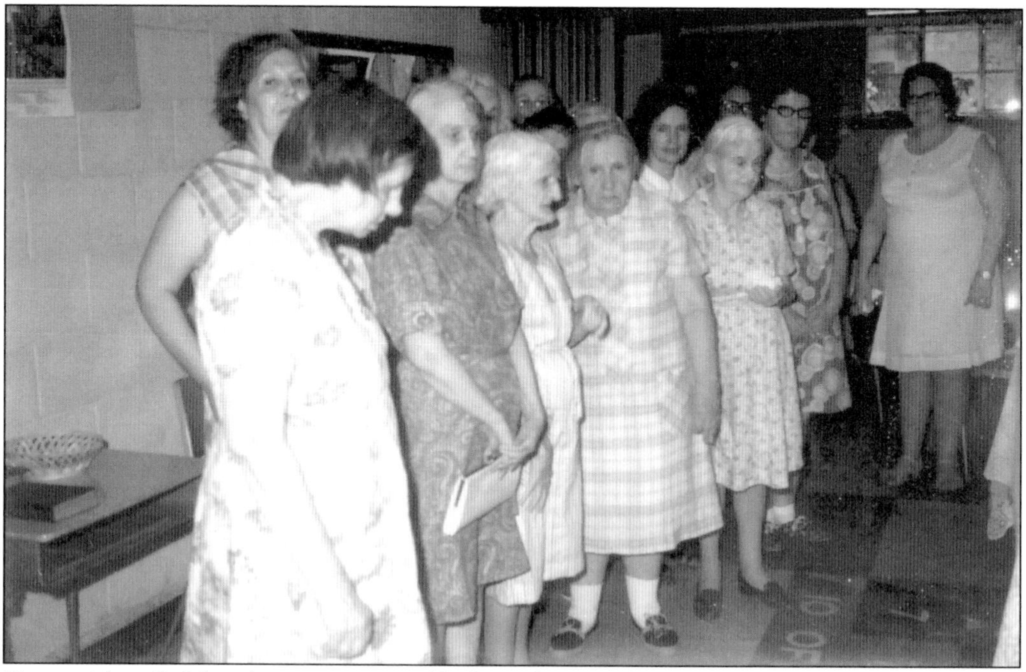

Here unidentified female patients assemble for a photograph. Patients and volunteers interacted seamlessly at Dixmont. One resocialization program met every Tuesday night and taught patients necessary life skills such as writing their names, learning other peoples' names, and dressing themselves. Volunteers like Dottie Lou and Lamon Forrester, Wil McSteen, and Tom Ceraso all logged approximately 1,000 volunteer hours each.

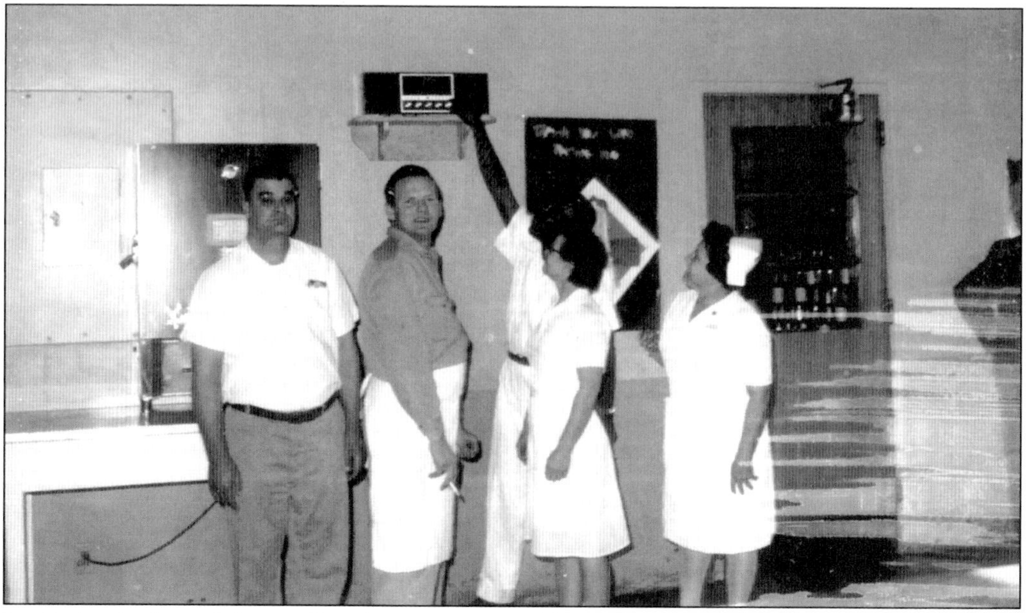

Declining budgets did not allow for luxuries, but Dixmont's supporters always found a way to come through for the hospital. This photograph commemorates the donation of a new radio to the dietary department in 1968. Then only identified person in the photograph is a man named Charles, a dietary employee, turning on the radio.

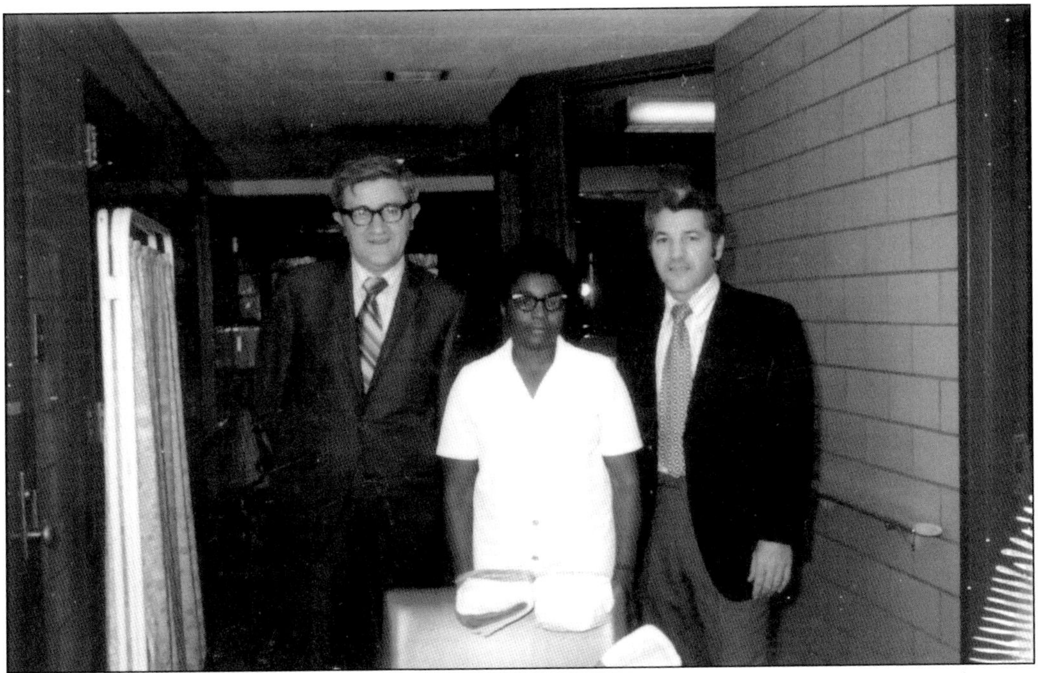

This unidentified nurse's aide, center, poses for a photograph on the first floor of the Hutchinson Building with representatives of Local 1211 Steelworkers, who donated a potty chair and supplies to Dixmont in 1972.

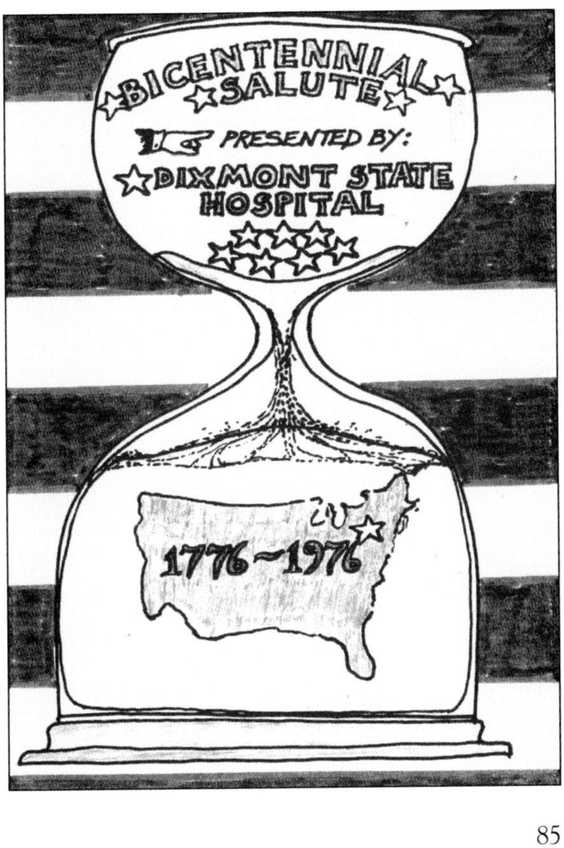

Major events of the outside world were not lost on those confined to Dixmont's majestic isolation. Staff ensured that holidays such as the Fourth of July were observed. Major historical events such as the moon landing and the bicentennial of the United States also were observed. This cover is from a program celebrating the bicentennial. (Courtesy Leroy Egan)

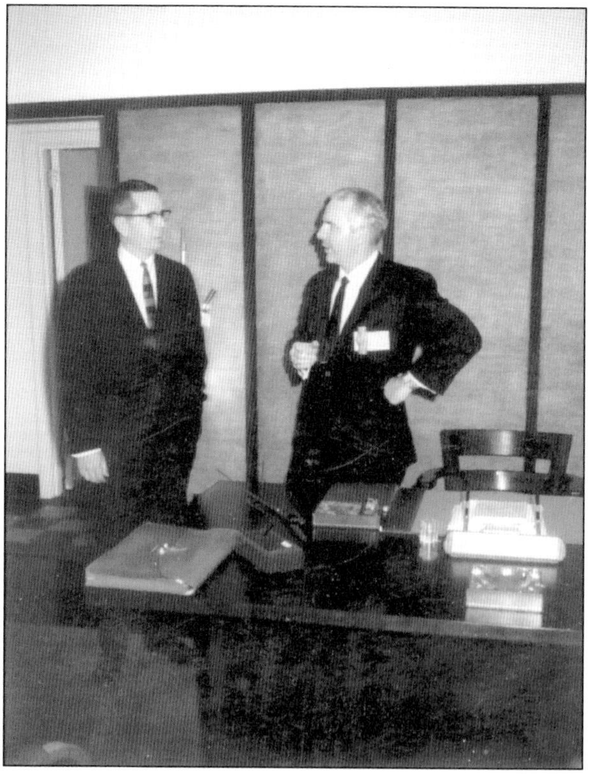

Despite growing adversity from the state, Dr. Robert Weimer continued his efforts to keep Dixmont vibrant. He instituted changes that increased the hospital's value—and incidentally, made it harder to destroy. These changes, such as accreditation and historic landmark status, all came under his tenure.

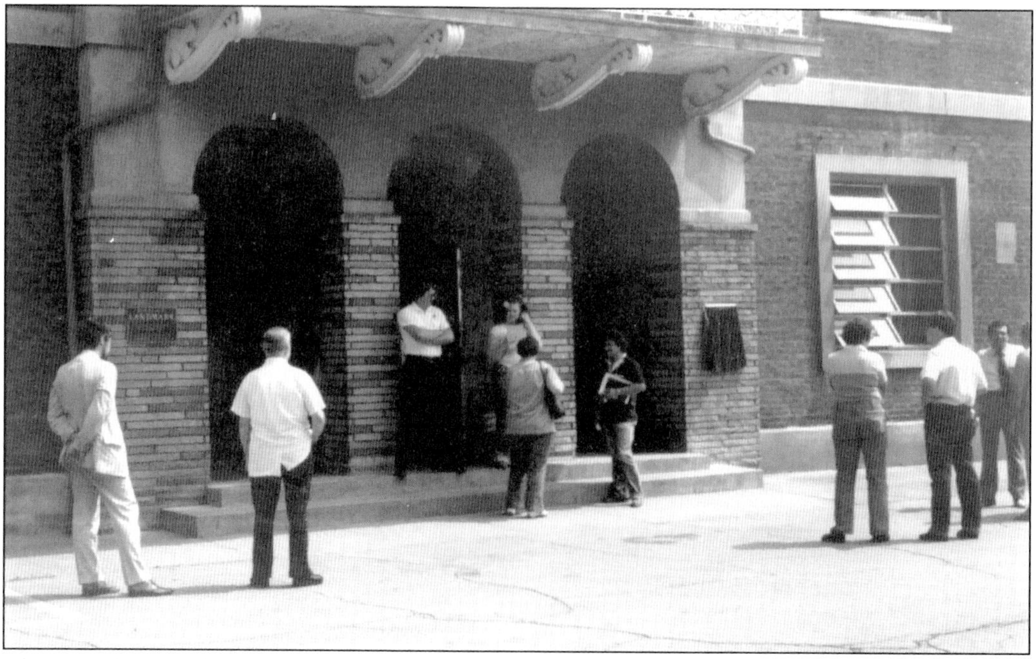

The unveiling of the National Register of Historic Places plaque on July 8, 1981, was a day of celebration. Here Dr. Leroy Egan stands on the far left. Jack Lennon, chief of security, stands with his arms folded in the center. The plaque is covered with a purple velvet curtain on the far right arch.

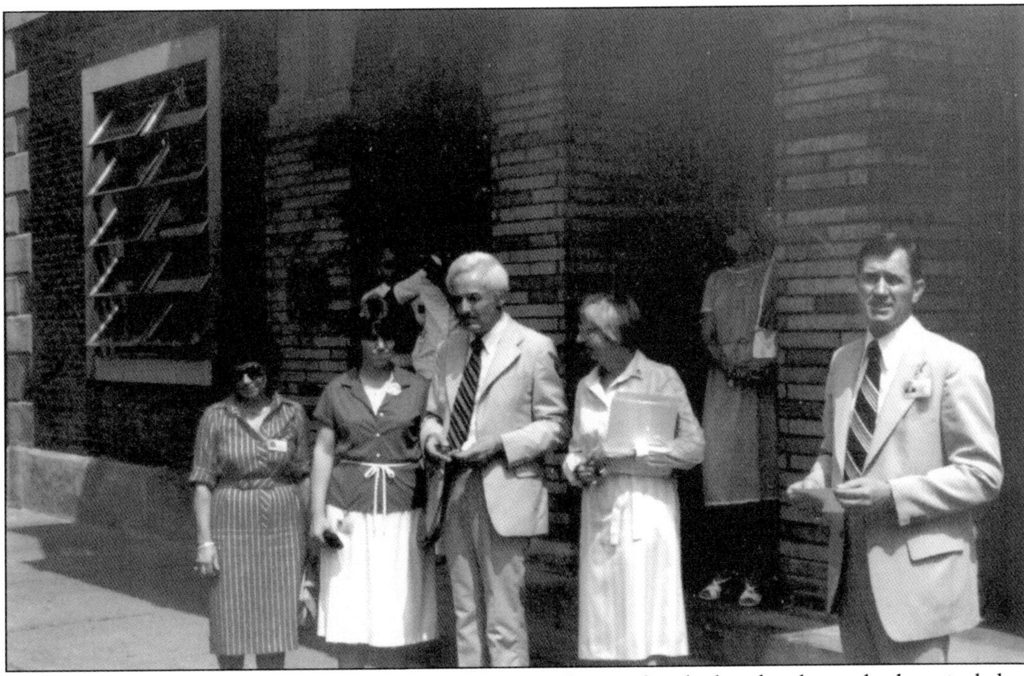

Despite being phased out by the state, Dixmont employees fought hard to keep the hospital they loved open. Part of that strategy was historical designation. Here Dr. Frank Lackner (center) with a group of unidentified people stands in front of Reed Hall during the landmark celebration for the building. (Courtesy Tracy Ferguson.)

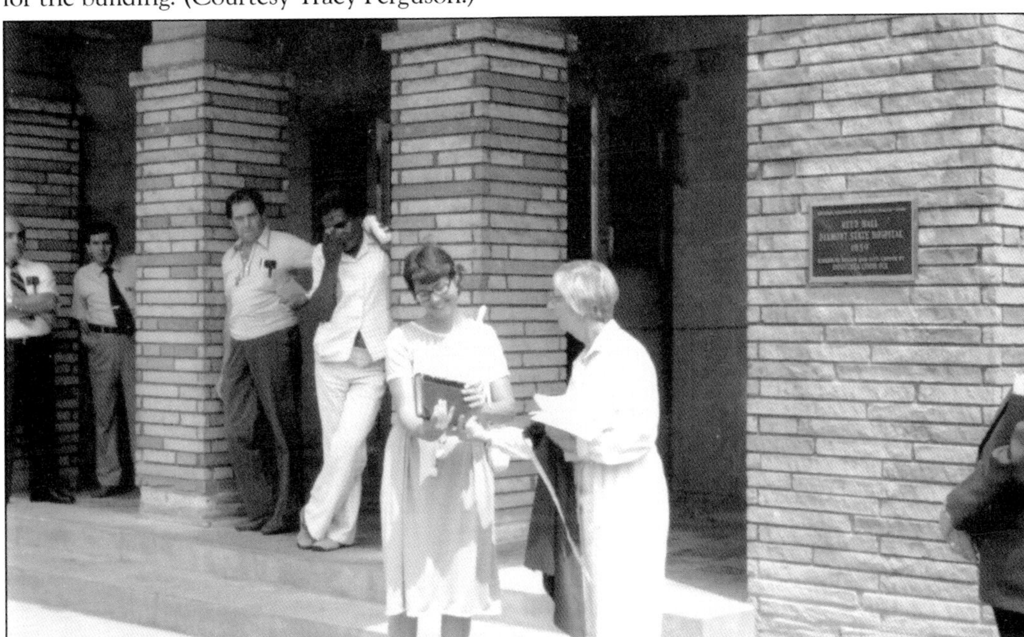

Beryl Randy Johnson, chairman of the Dixmont Historical Committee, shares a copy of an early Dixmont manager's report with Anica Reed Smith, great-great-granddaughter of Dr. Joseph Allison Reed. Reed served from 1862 until he was forced to take a leave of absence because of illness. He died on November 6, 1884. (Courtesy Tracy Ferguson.)

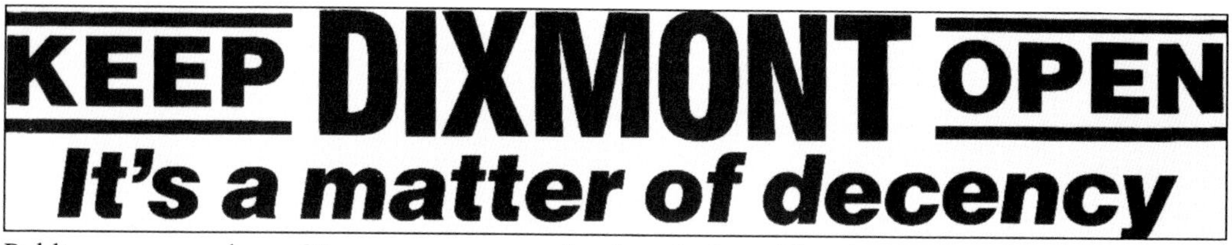

Public outcry to keep Dixmont open was loud and clear. This bumper sticker, originally in fluorescent orange, captures the feeling of support against Dixmont's demise and the general trend of deinstitutionalization that started in the 1950s. Similar efforts kept other hospitals alive on borrowed time, such as Woodville. However, even Woodville became subject to demolition in 2000 after a long vacancy. (Courtesy Helen Wolf.)

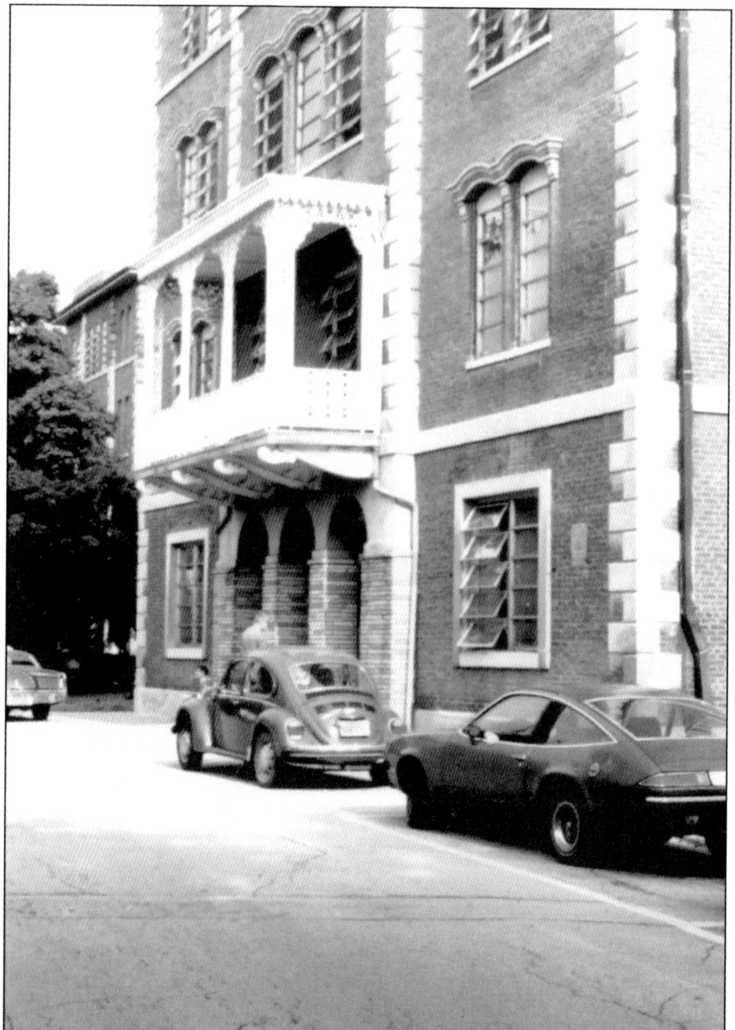

On June 30, 1984, Dixmont's doors were closed and locked for good. Despite ambitions to better the hospital with an activities building, swimming pool, and community outreach programs, Dixmont finally had outlived its usefulness in the eyes of the state. Its remaining patients were transferred to Mayview and Woodville State Hospitals. The move was projected to save the state $12.5 million annually.

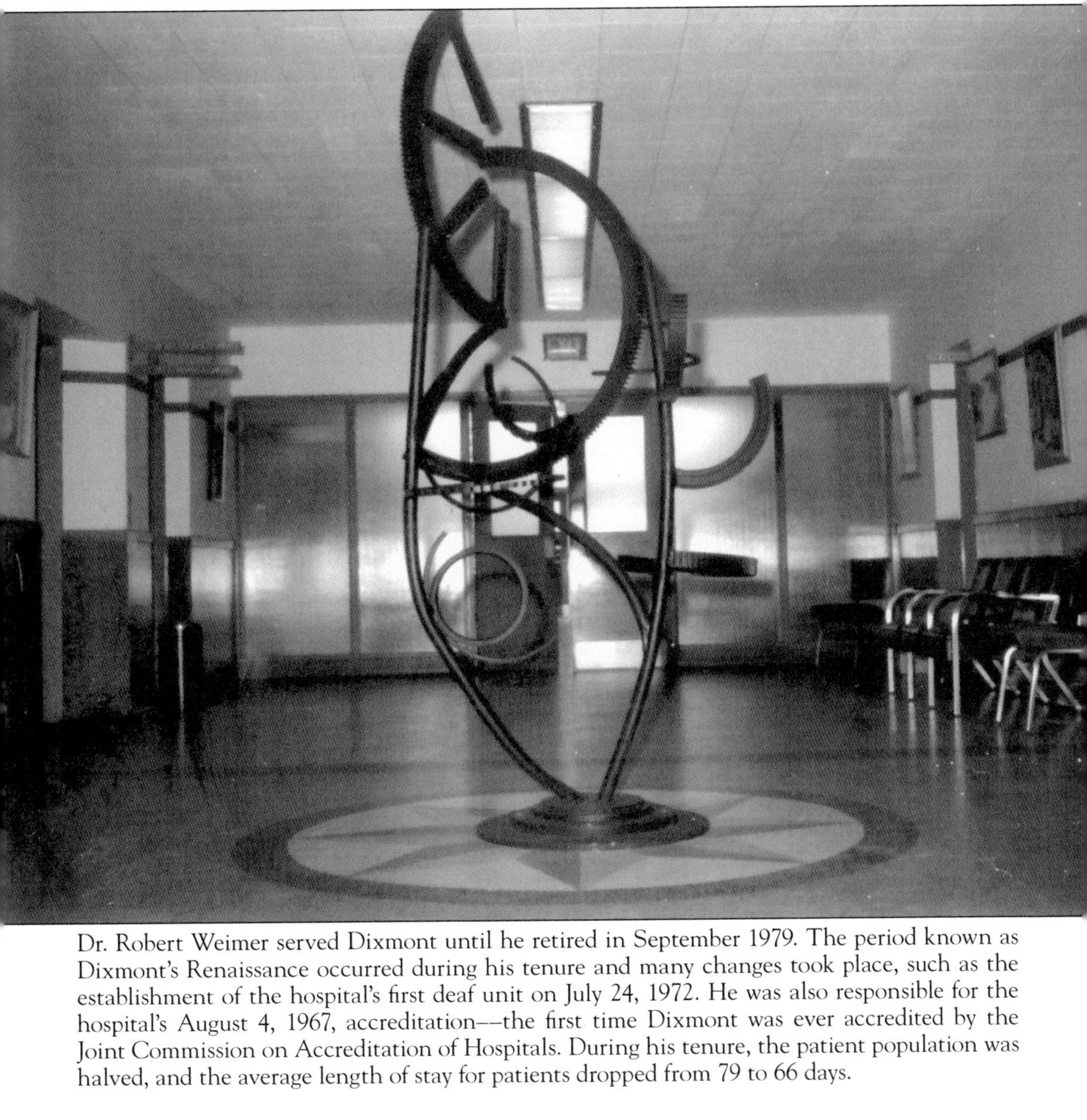

Dr. Robert Weimer served Dixmont until he retired in September 1979. The period known as Dixmont's Renaissance occurred during his tenure and many changes took place, such as the establishment of the hospital's first deaf unit on July 24, 1972. He was also responsible for the hospital's August 4, 1967, accreditation—the first time Dixmont was ever accredited by the Joint Commission on Accreditation of Hospitals. During his tenure, the patient population was halved, and the average length of stay for patients dropped from 79 to 66 days.

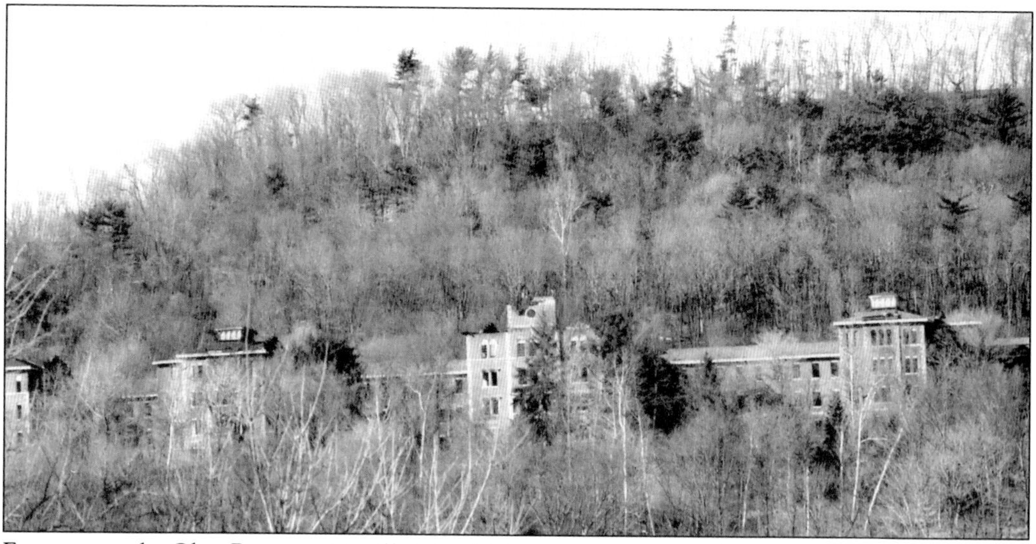

From across the Ohio River, on Neville Island, Dixmont appears to blend in with its surroundings. The property was heavily wooded and became overgrown after Dixmont's closing. During this time, Dixmont became a property in search of a buyer. A county jail was proposed and reviled by Dixmont's neighboring communities. After strong opposition, Dixmont was removed from the list of potential locations, and on October 3, 1989, Allegheny County commissioners officially announced that Dixmont would not be the site of a $50 million jail. The property again sat dormant. By June 25, 1998, the minimum bid for the property was lowered from $1.5 million to $596,900 in order to entice more competition by developers.

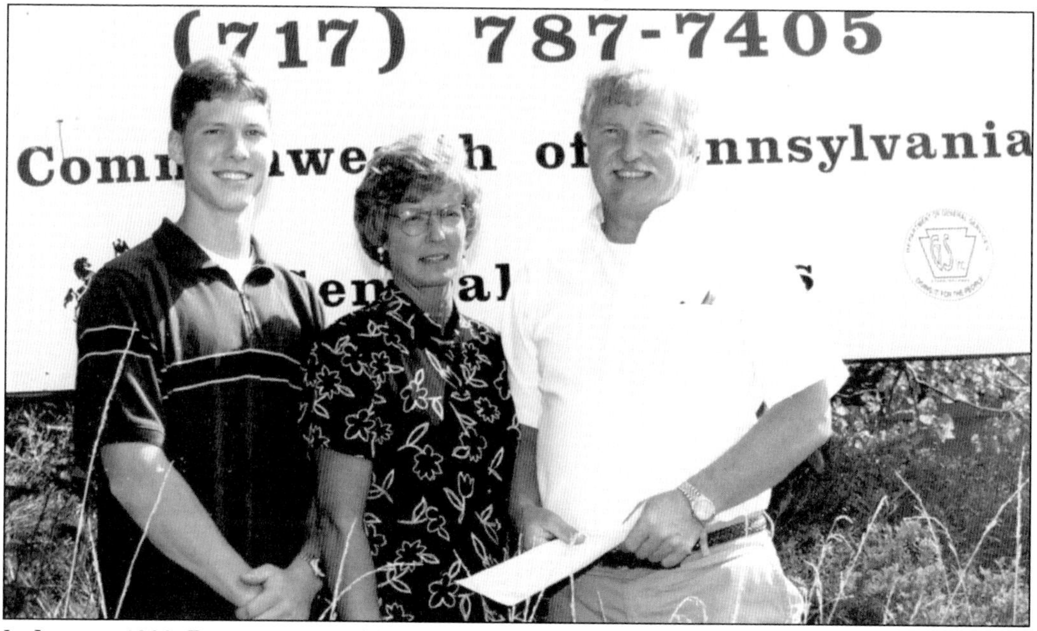

In January 1999, Dixmont was sold to Ralph Stroyne, far right, shown here with his son, Tim, and wife, Carole. The purchase price was $757,000. Stroyne's father, Bill, was a butcher at Dixmont and his uncle was a Dixmont mechanic. The family has a farm near the property. Today the Stroynes own and operate the Cammarata Building––the last remaining structure from Dixmont. (Courtesy of Connie Rankin/the Citizen.)

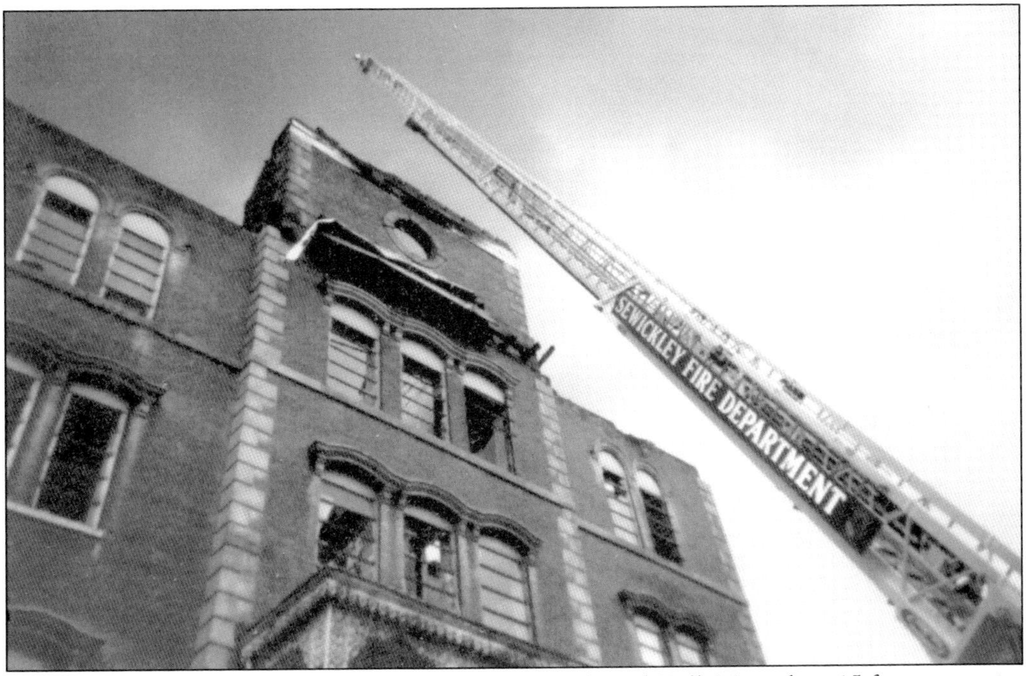

On June 2, 1995, an enormous fire gutted the center of Reed Hall. More than 15 fire companies responded to the blaze. Here is one of the Sewickley Fire Department's ladder trucks at the scene. Arson was determined to be the cause of the fire, which started in the hospital's chapel. (Courtesy Zachary Stauffer.)

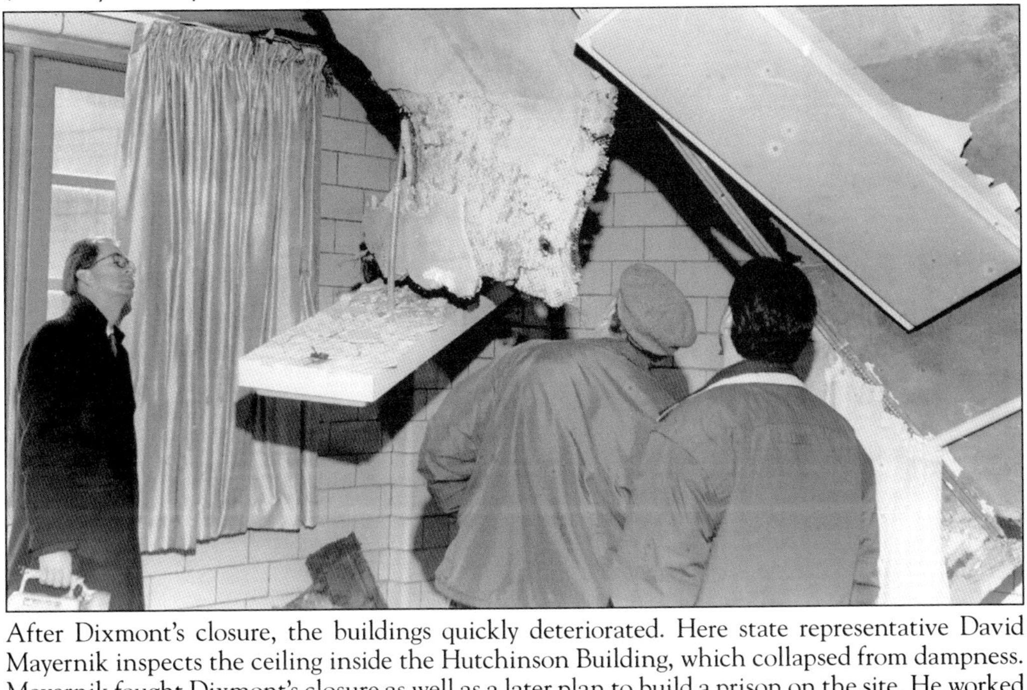

After Dixmont's closure, the buildings quickly deteriorated. Here state representative David Mayernik inspects the ceiling inside the Hutchinson Building, which collapsed from dampness. Mayernik fought Dixmont's closure as well as a later plan to build a prison on the site. He worked to find developers for the site and supported the desires of the community to get the property back on the tax rolls. (Courtesy Connie Rankin/the Citizen.)

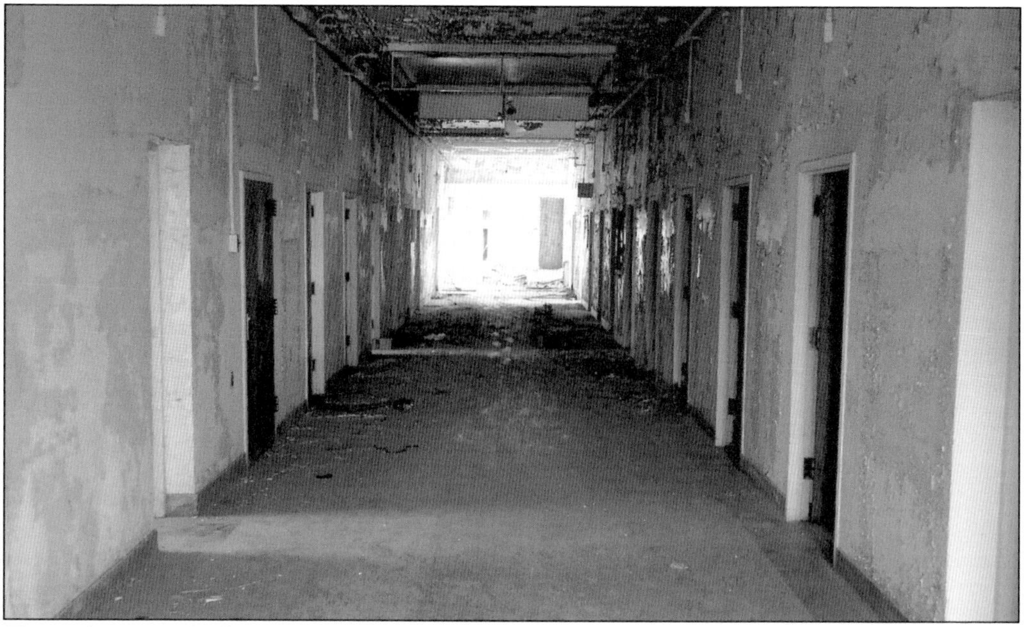

Shown here is a hallway in Reed Hall. This hallway could easily be any hallway within the building. Each ward had a set of rooms, nurses' station with mini-pharmacies, and lounging areas. Most wards had bulletin boards or murals to break up the wall space. Dixmont's wards were divided by gender and municipal locations––Beaver and Lawrence Counties.

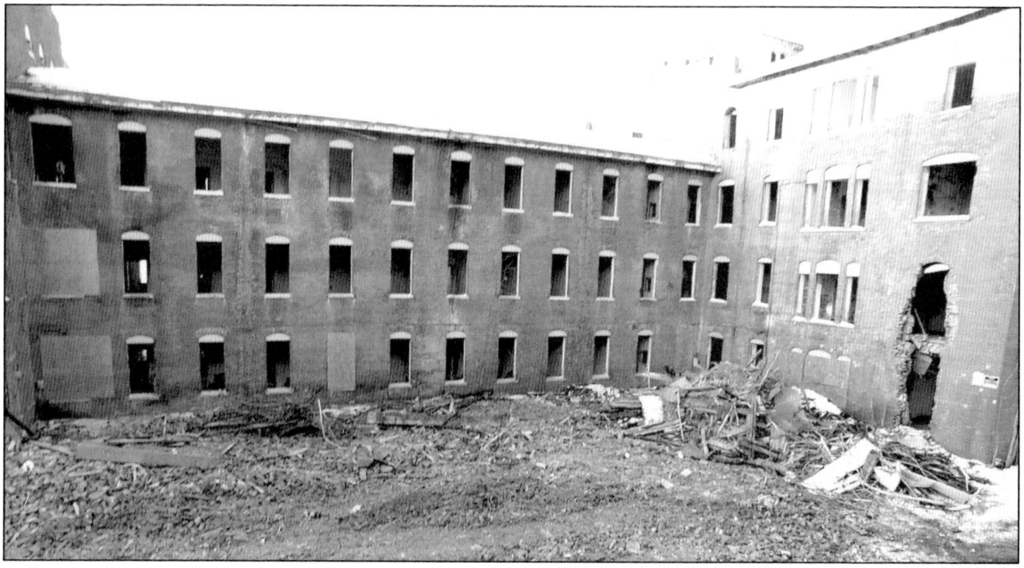

This perspective is from the dietary building facing the back of Reed Hall. The stark view with windows broken out is what gave Dixmont some of its spooky appeal. Local radio stations would spend Halloween night on the premises, and local ghost hunters claimed to have found evidence of otherworldly entities, posting their findings on their Web sites. However, the fact is that once sold to the Stroyne family, vandals broke virtually every window in the building. The few remaining bars on the windows were sold for scrap, as were the copper and other metals in the building such as doorknobs, lock sets, and so on. The end result was an extremely bare, desolate shell of a building.

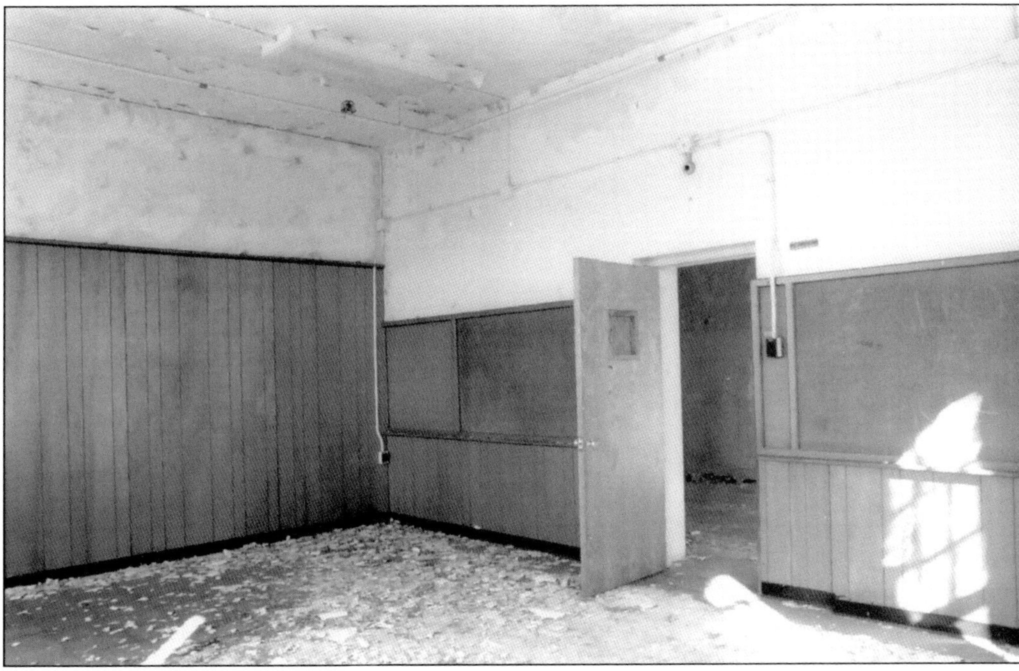

This classroom was on the third floor of Reed Hall. Dixmont staff held adult basic education programs for its patients. These classes were administered by the Allegheny County Intermediate Unit, which provided counselors, teachers, and aides. Hospital aides also served as teachers' aides. Patients could learn math, reading, and social skills.

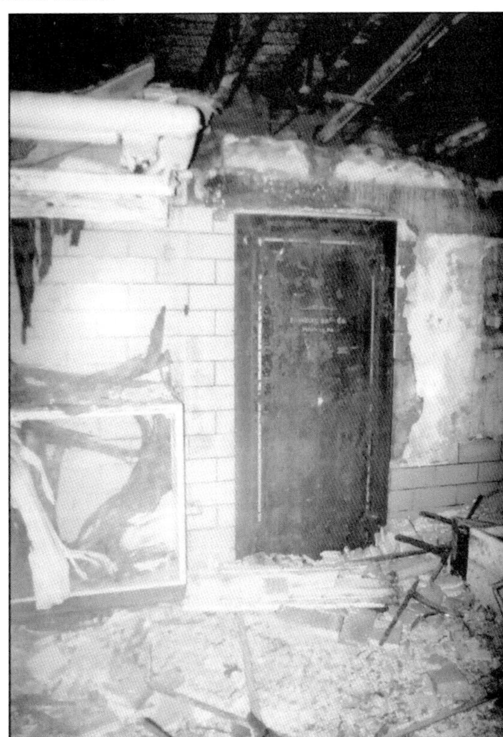

Beneath Reed Hall was the old pharmacy. In 1971, the pharmacy, located behind this steel door, was transferred to the first floor of the Lawrence Unit, and this area was used for archives. Shortly after, in 1973, the situation was reversed, and the vault held the drugs for the institution once more.

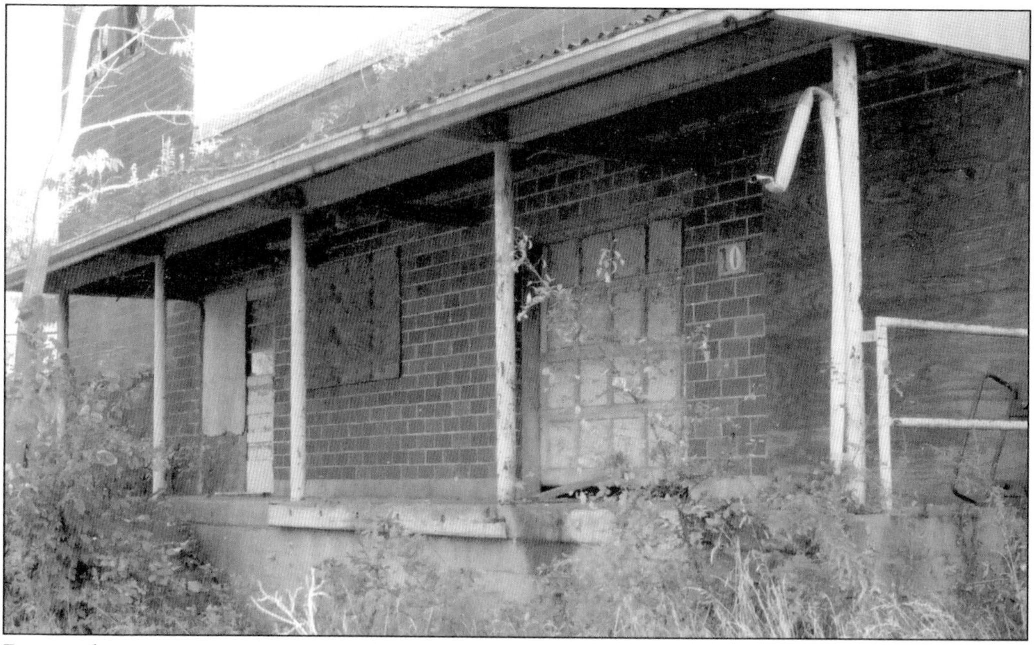

Despite having its own laundry building, state budget cuts required Dixmont's laundry to be done at Woodville State Hospital in Collier Township. This arrangement was not practical, and employees recorded many shortcomings of the program ranging from collection to production in the Quality Assurance Committee minutes.

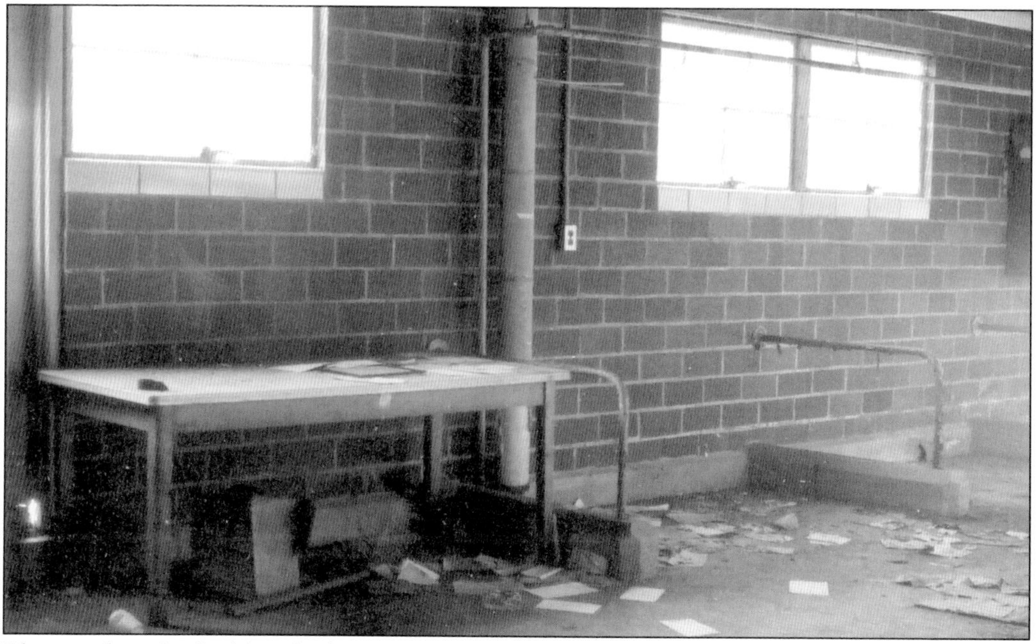

The new laundry building had one of the longest-working Dixmont employees, George Fleck, who was assigned head laundryman in 1954. The last of a dying breed at state hospitals, Fleck originally started under the superintendence of Henry Hutchinson as a swineherd. He lived on the property for more than 20 years, after which the state started phasing out the practice of having staff live on hospital grounds.

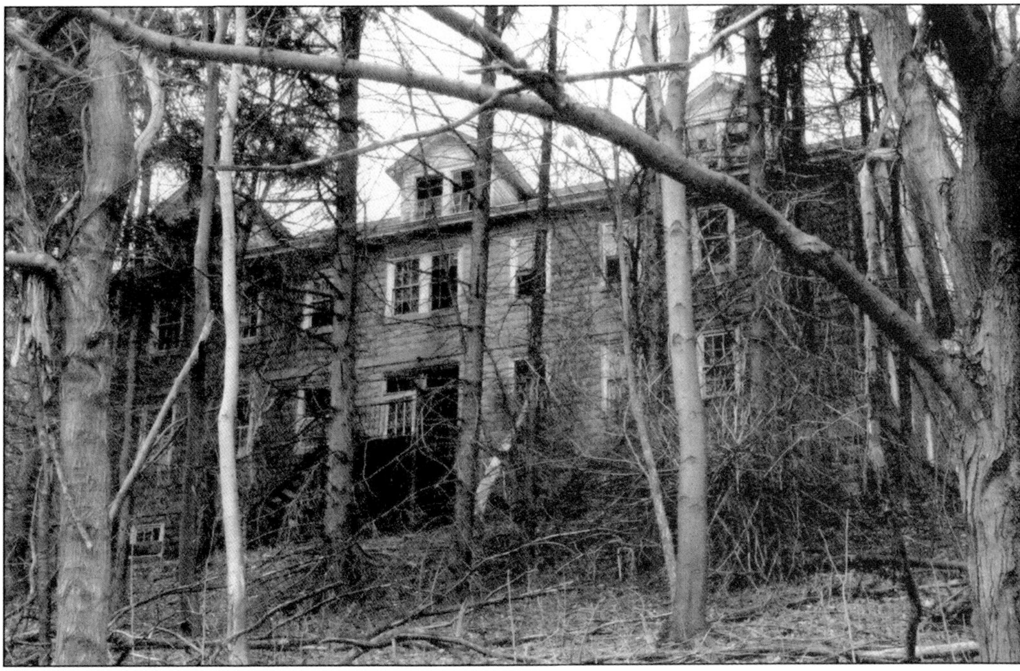

The industrial arts building was one of the newer buildings on the property. Built of cast concrete in 1933, the two-and-a-half-story building was passed over for historic preservation surveys of the property. The industrial arts department provided "an immense amount of work done," superintendent Henry Hutchinson wrote in 1934.

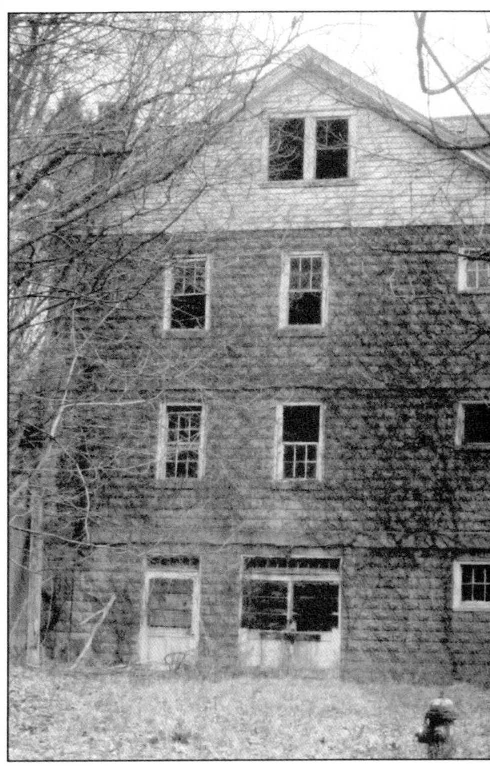

Items manufactured by the industrial arts department were varied and ranged from aprons and awnings to bed sheets, trellises, coats, overalls, mattresses, and pillows. The department also mended hundreds of pairs of pants, vests, and shoes each year. The department also upholstered the hospital's sleighs and stretcher pads.

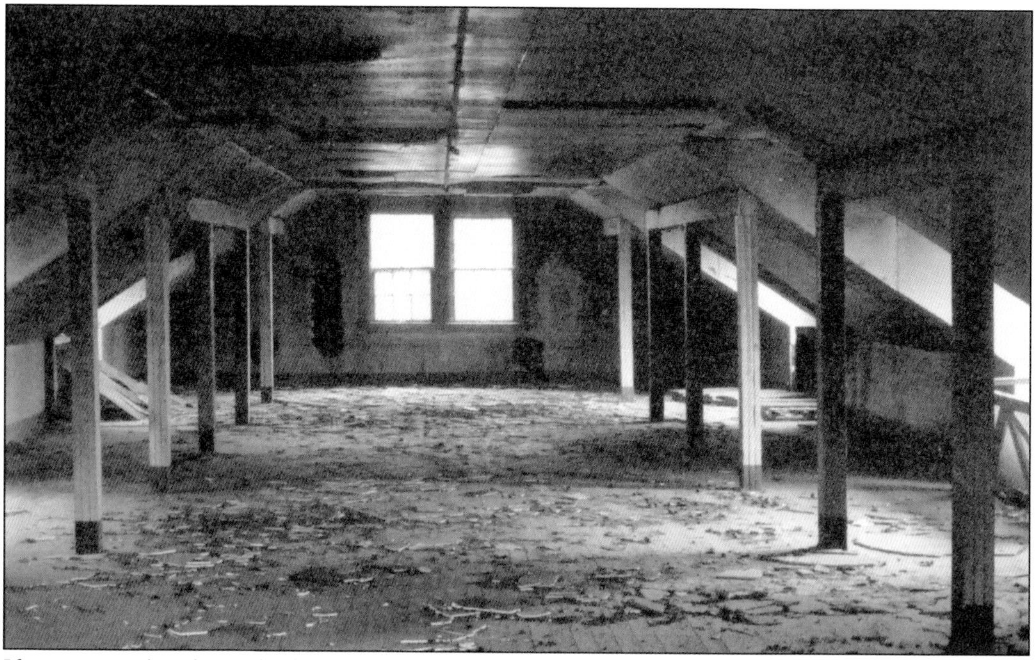

If it was made of wood, chances are it passed through the industrial arts department. The department refinished hundreds of pieces of furniture for the hospital, including birdhouses, chairs, clocks, pianos, refrigerators, desks, folding screens, and picture frames, of which 186 were refinished in 1933 alone. Nearly 70 more were refinished the following year.

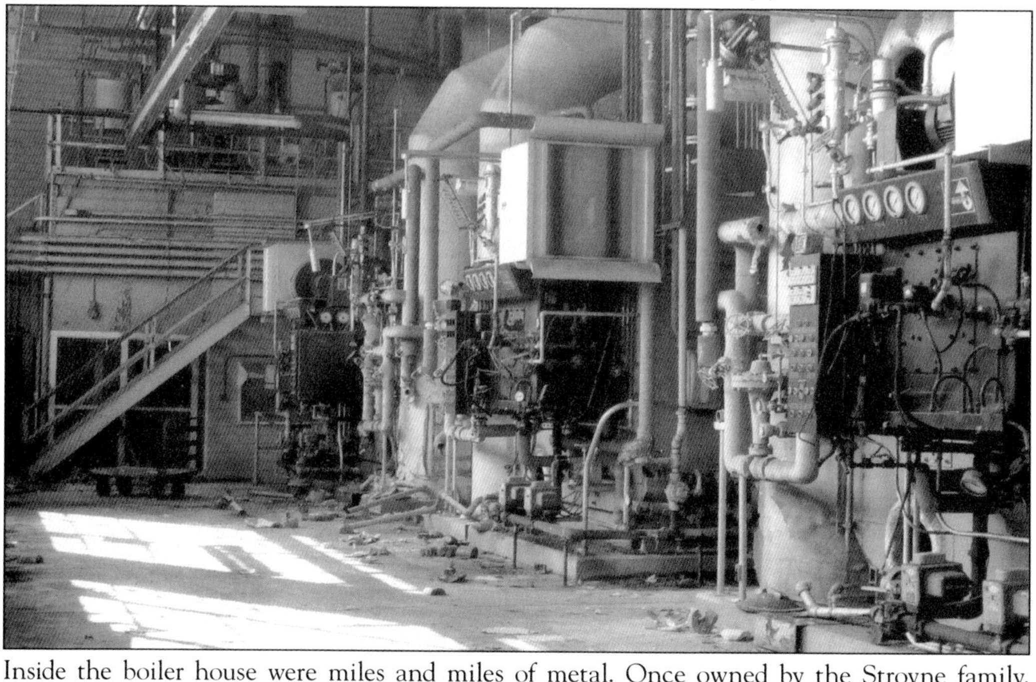

Inside the boiler house were miles and miles of metal. Once owned by the Stroyne family, scavengers purchased as much valuable stock as possible. The boiler house was connected to Reed Hall by a long concrete tunnel. The boiler house was upgraded to oil-burning on June 10, 1976. The project was completed by August 1977.

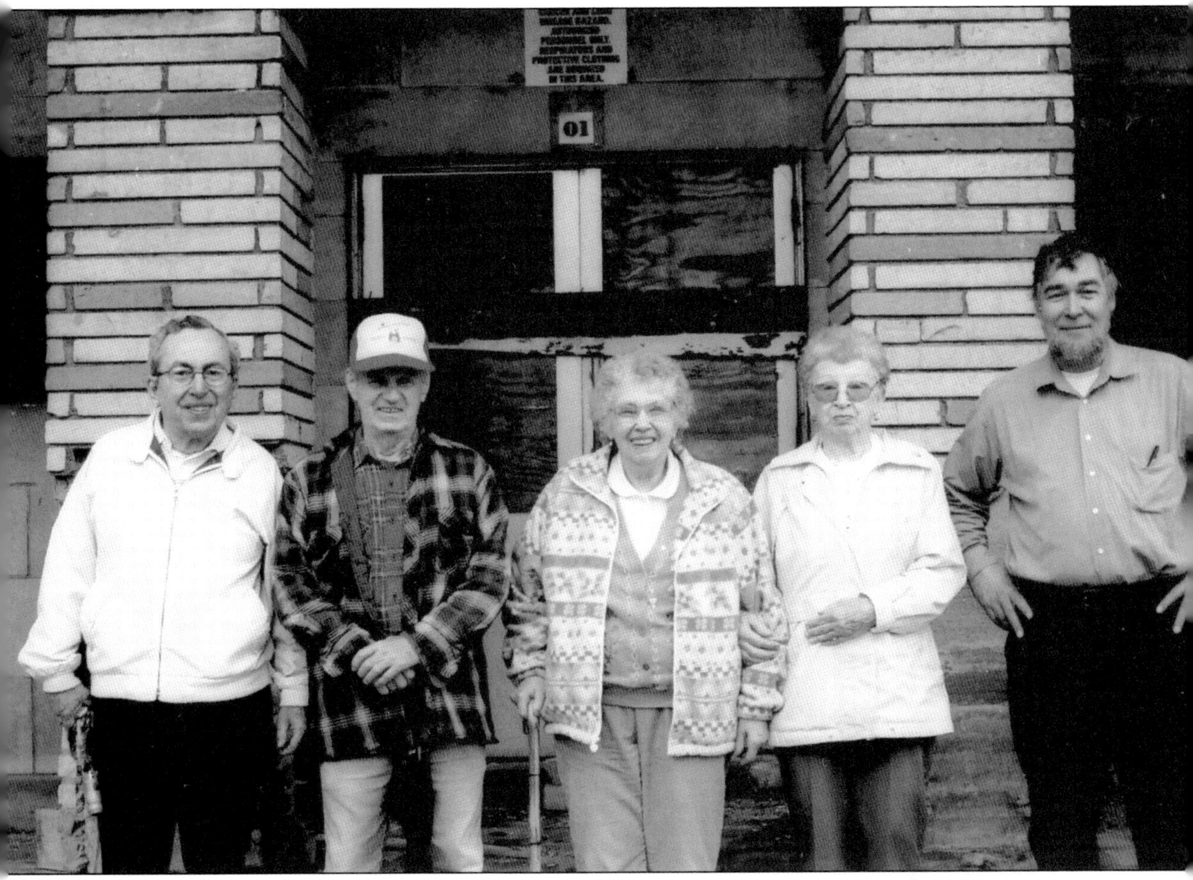

From left to right, Kirby Gould, Bill Wolf, Christine Turner, Dorothy Snyder, and Leroy Egan stand in front of Reed Hall. This was the last time they were on site together prior to Dixmont's demolition. Many of Dixmont's former employees are relieved that something is being done with the property simply because it pains them to see the buildings in such ruin.

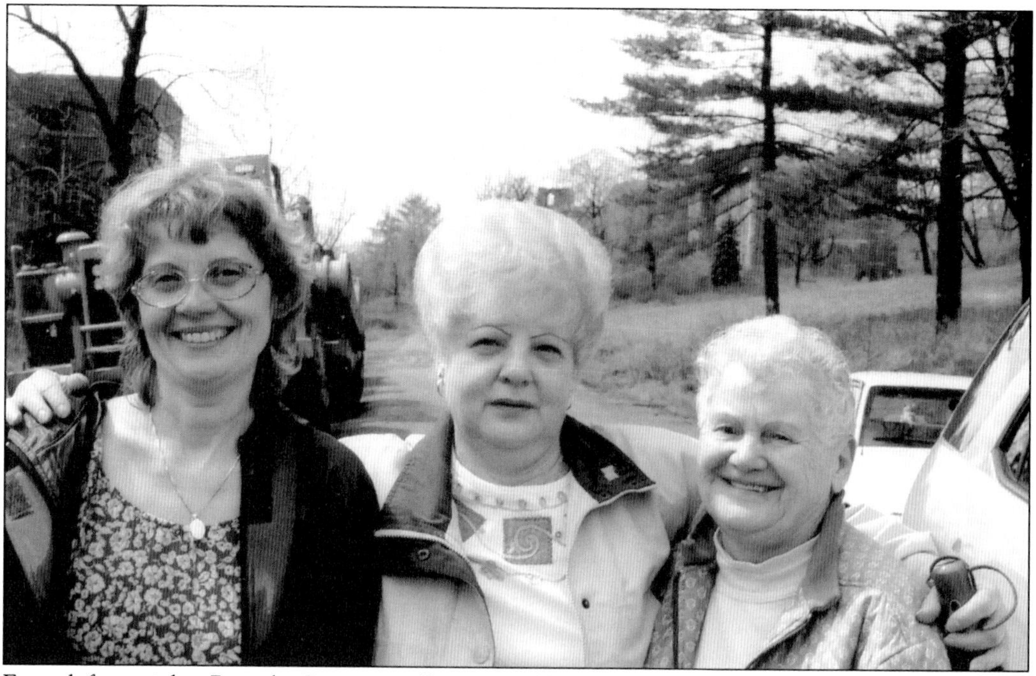

From left to right, Beverly Cummins (former staff nurse), Rose Glevicky, and an unidentified person stand in front of the Rosenzweig House. Behind them is a large excavator that sat dormant on site for months as a community group tried in vain to stop the Dixmont demolition.

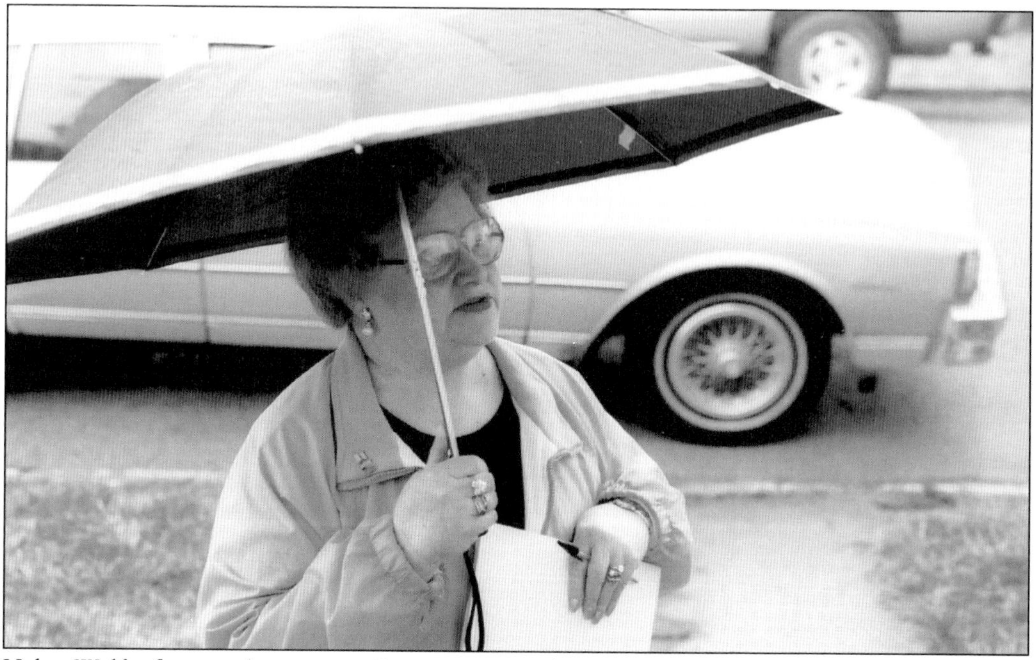

Helen Wolf reflects on her years at Dixmont as a volunteer coordinator. Even though more than two decades have passed since her time at Dixmont, Wolf is still volunteering on behalf of the hospital she loves by organizing the Dixmont reunions. She transferred to Woodville when Dixmont closed.

On Sunday January 6, 2002, more than 140 years after it was buried, Ralph Stroyne was able to find the cornerstone to Dixmont State Hospital. The stone lay nearly 12 feet below the ground level. Here an excavator operated by Jim Ott knocks the rock from the foundation. (Courtesy www.dixmontstate.com.)

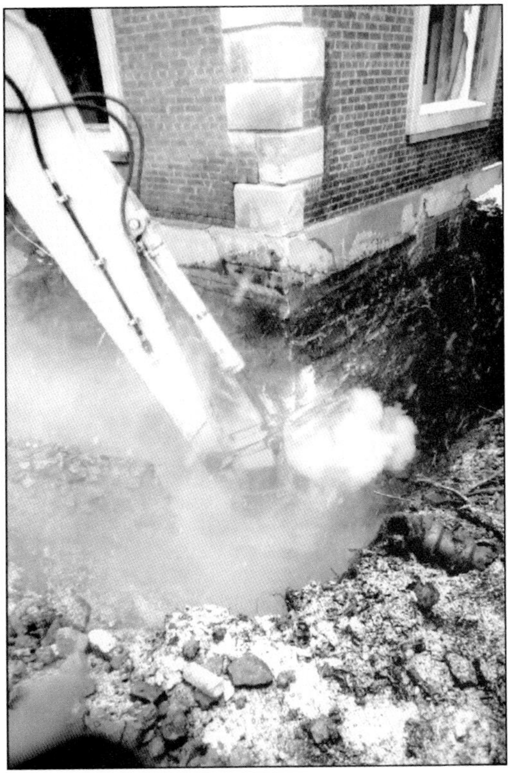

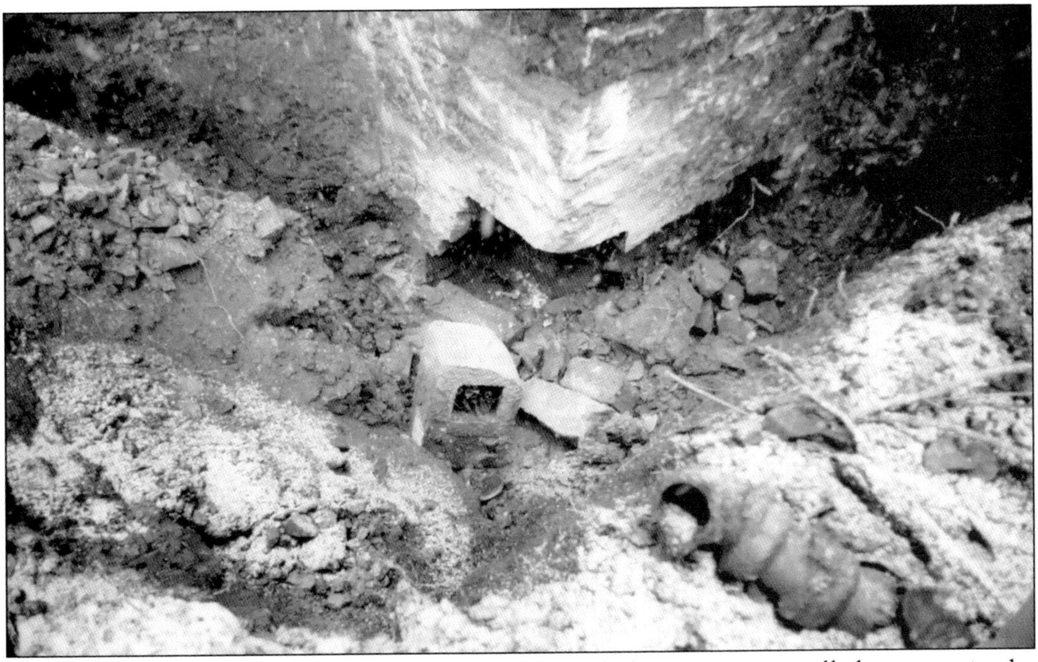

Once the smoke cleared, a simple stone with a hewn hole in its center rolled to a rest in the mud. Records show that the stone was quarried from locations on-site. Stroyne, who owns a large collection of Dixmont memorabilia, looked for the stone in various places over the years, leaving large holes in Reed Hall. (Courtesy www.dixmontstate.com.)

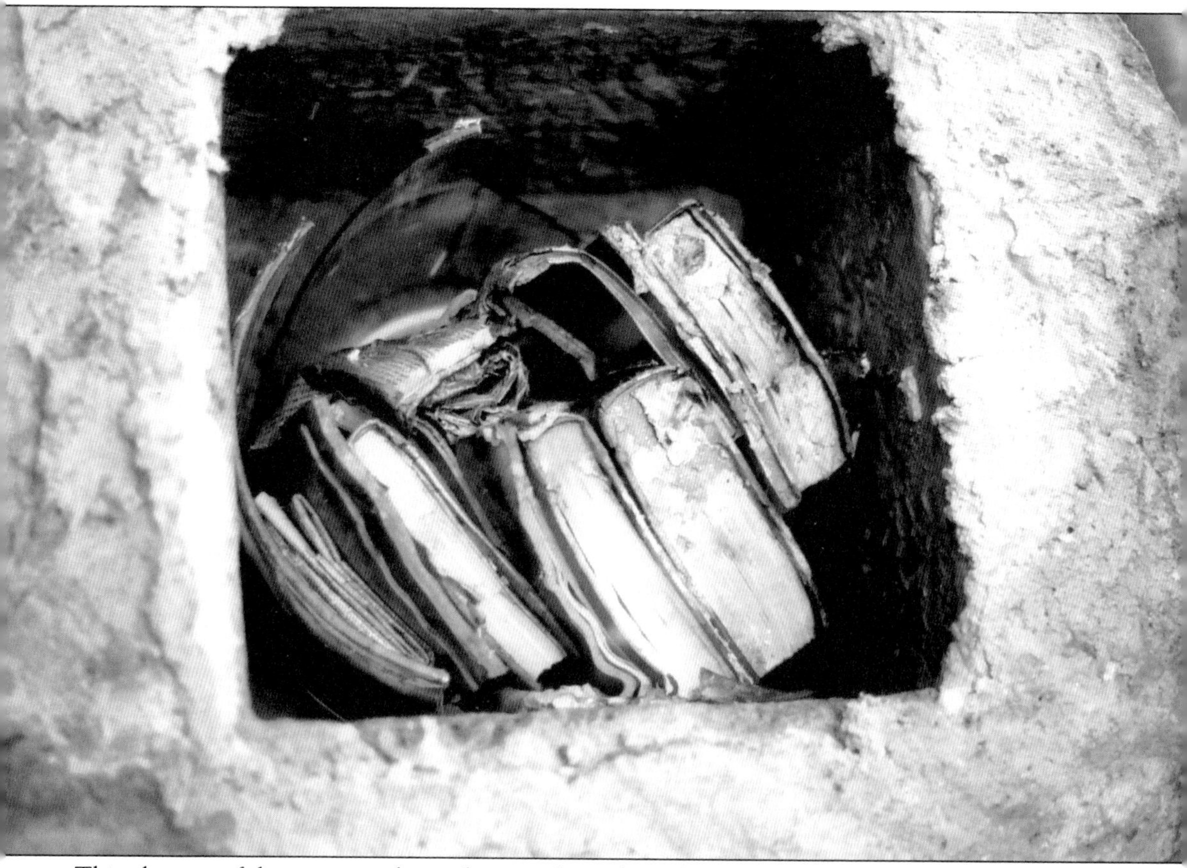

This close-up of the contents shows the waterlogged condition of the time capsule. The contents included *The Olden Time* by Neville B. Craig; the Pittsburgh directory, 1859; *Account of the Great Fire of 1845*; a letter from Dorothea Lynde Dix, which included the lyrics to a hymn written by M. M. R., a former patient; reports of the House of Refuge for 1859; a list of the members of the Pennsylvania legislature; all of the Pittsburgh dailies, New York newspapers, and other miscellaneous news records; 1859 Almanac; Dix's 1855 report to the legislature; and a bronze medal of Allegheny County Agricultural Society. (Courtesy www.dixmontstate.com.)

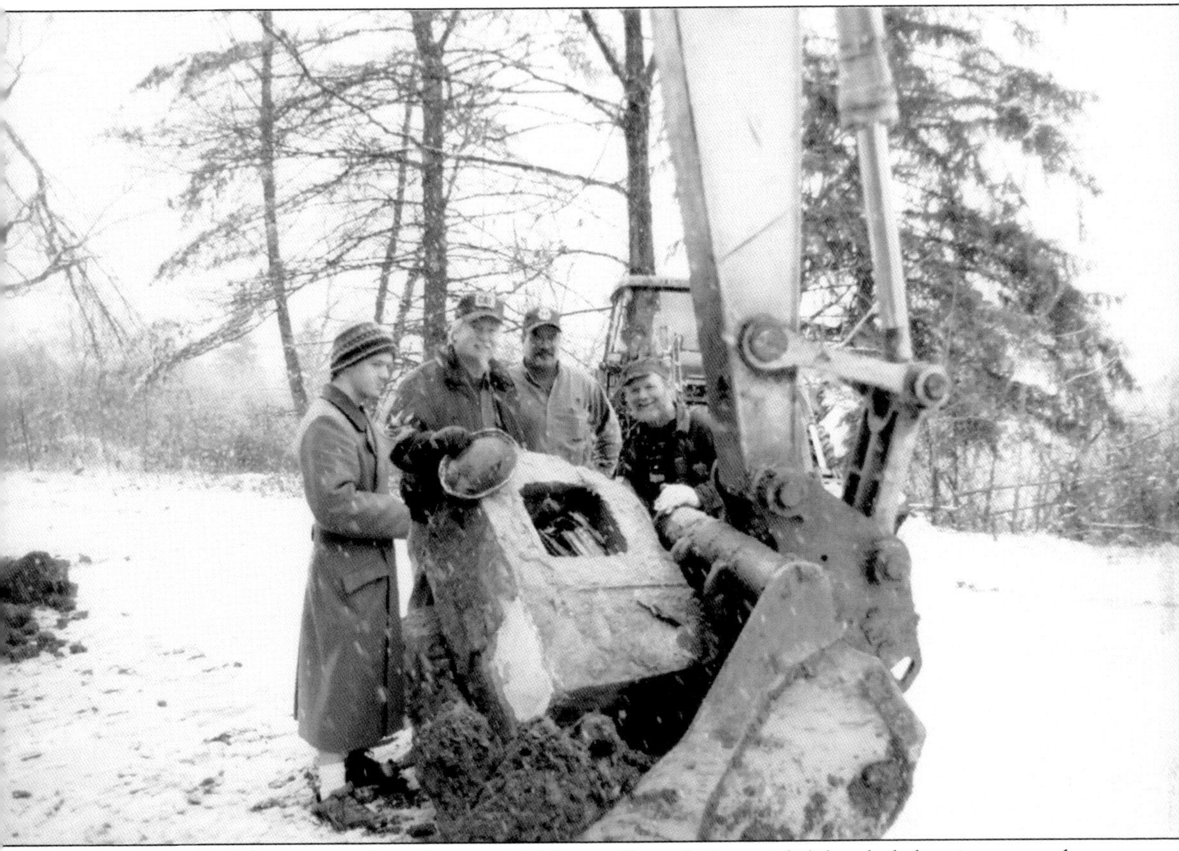

Zak Jones, Ralph Stroyne, Jim Ott, and Al Jones (from left to right) hauled the time capsule to the surface. Today the stone is a landscape feature on the Stroyne farm. The contents of the time capsule were taken to the Carnegie Library by the author to determine if its contents were worth salvaging. Because the contents of the capsule were comprised of items already in the Carnegie's collection, it was deemed valueless. It is now in the possession of the Ben Avon Area Historical Association. (Courtesy www.dixmontstate.com.)

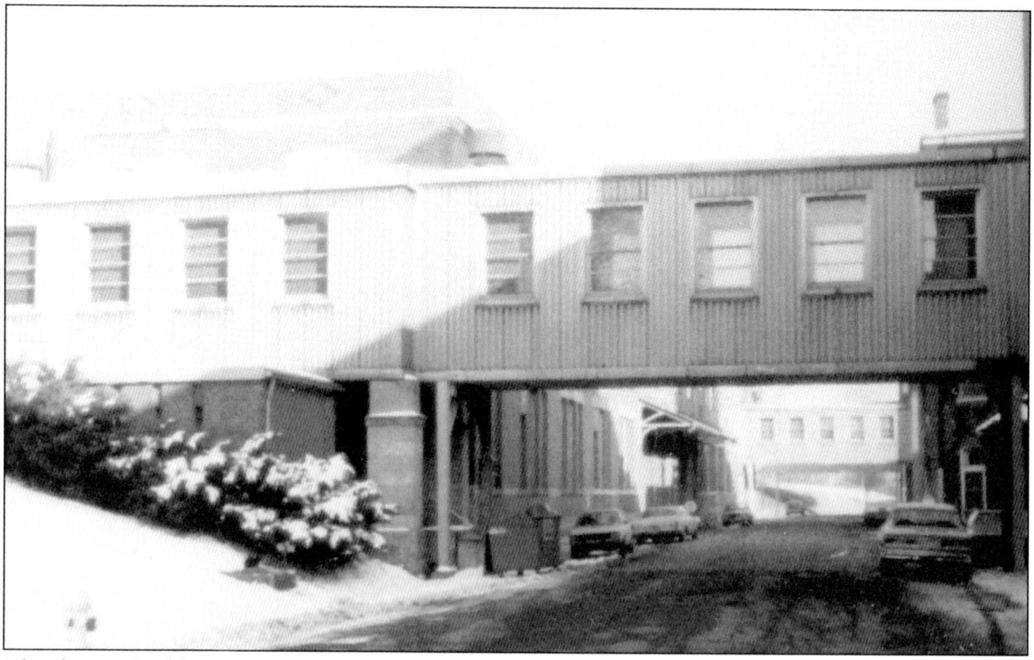

The dietary building was attached to Reed Hall by means of several pedestrian walkways. These walkways bridged over a driveway that ran behind Reed Hall and offered access to the garage doors on the lower level of the dietary building, where deliveries were made. The lower level of the dietary building also housed the refrigeration equipment.

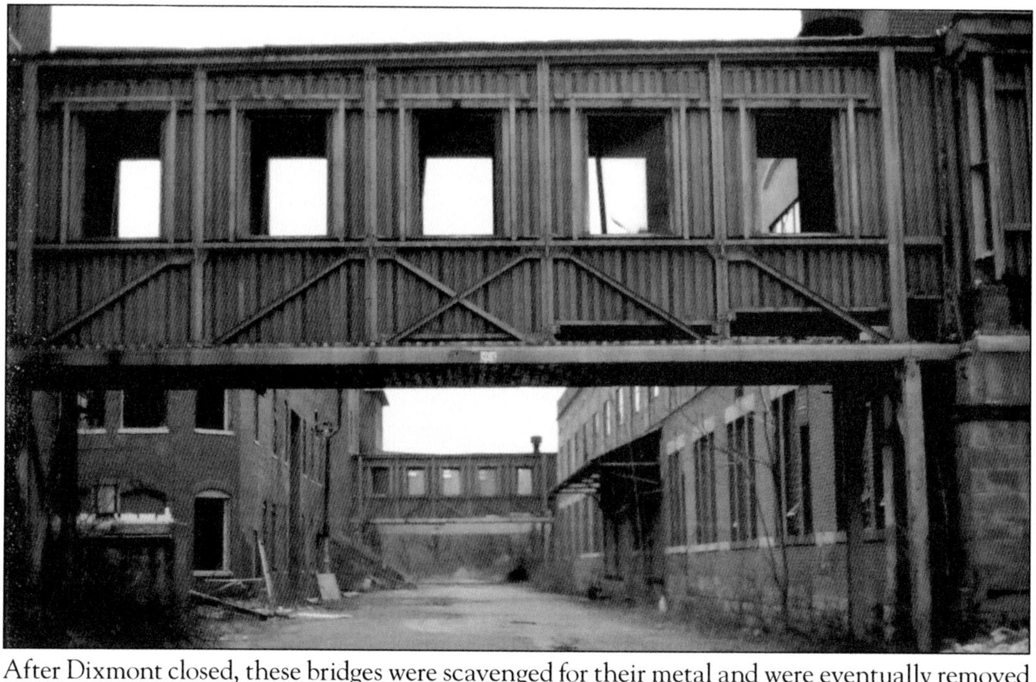

After Dixmont closed, these bridges were scavenged for their metal and were eventually removed completely. The bridges were rebuilt in 1969, and their enclosed design was improved upon. In all, there were four bridges branching out from Reed Hall—two to access the dietary building and two for fire escape.

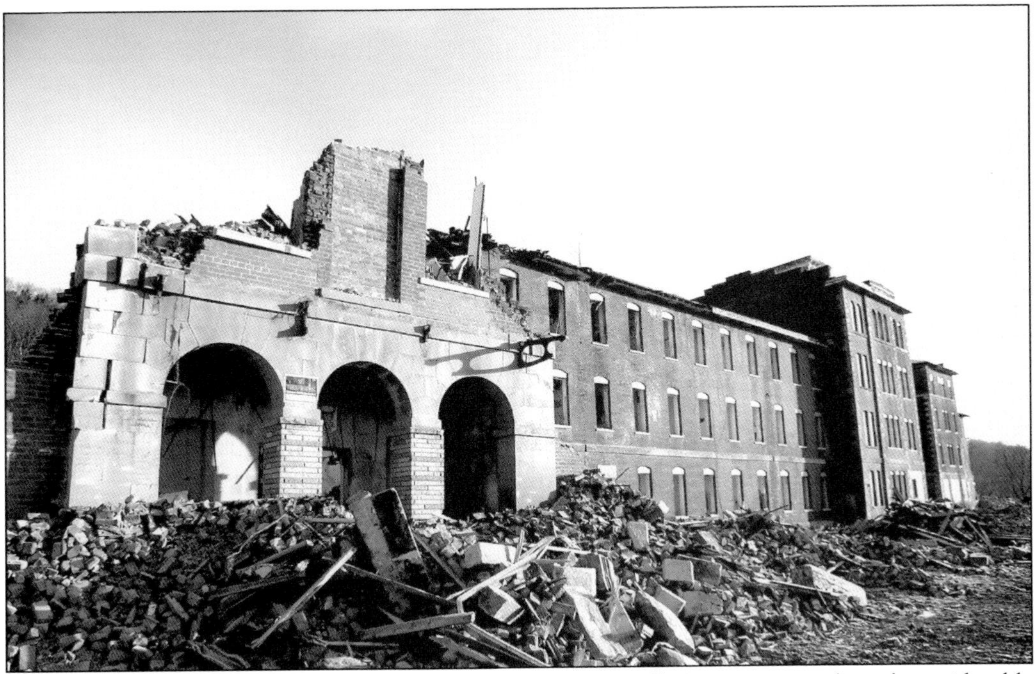

By February 2006, there was virtually nothing left of Reed Hall. Construction slowed considerably on April 26, when a morning blasting error collapsed a rocky hillside down onto Route 65. The collapse resulted in traffic stoppages for the rest of the day. Blasting later resumed on the site.

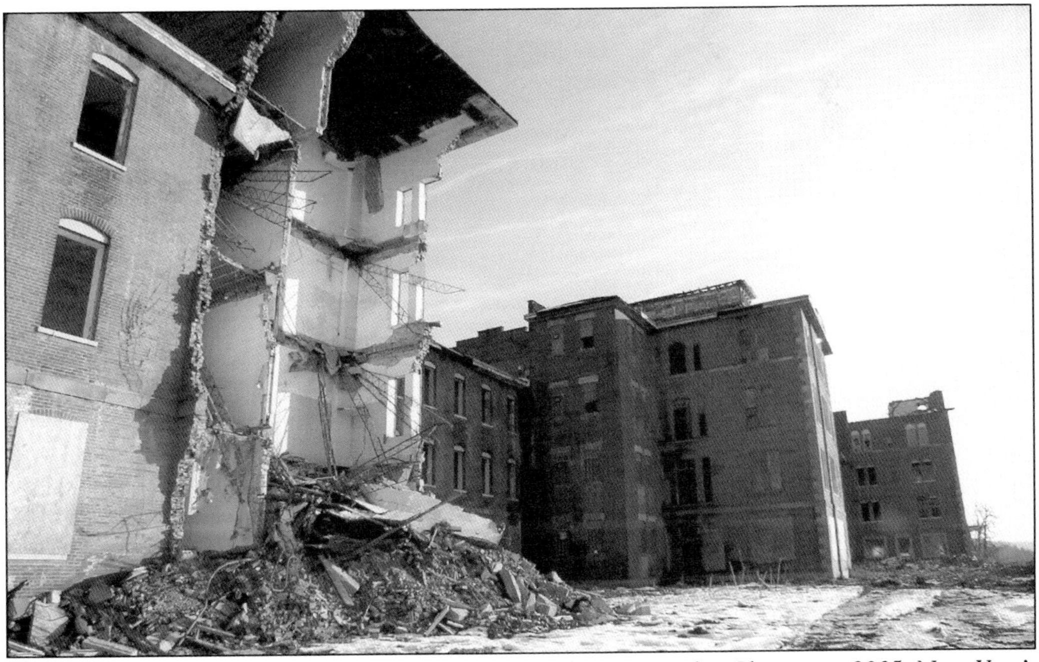

The demolition of Reed Hall was swift and carried out over the Christmas 2005–New Year's 2006 holiday season, when this photograph was taken. Demolition started on the Lawrence County ward section. The sweeping back of the Kirkbride design is apparent from this angle. The main entrance to Reed Hall is on the far right of the frame.

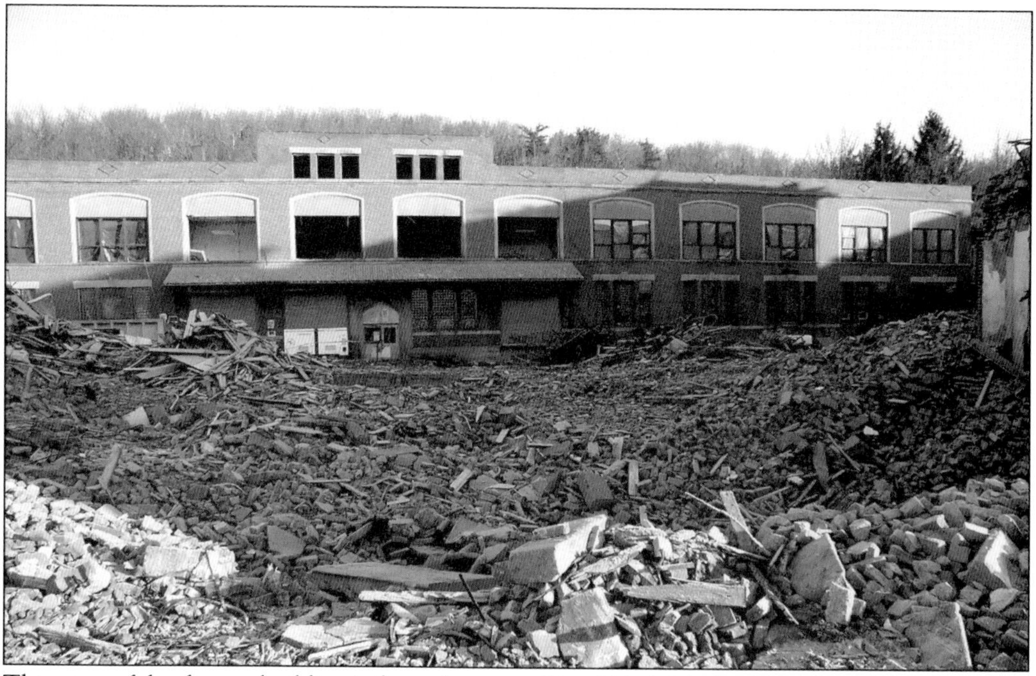

This view of the dietary building is from the rear of Reed Hall. Much of this area was demolished after a 1995 fire in Reed Hall. The bottom half of the dietary building was used for storage of abandoned beds and miscellaneous items left behind. Some of the headboards and drawers had personal belongings, such as sticker books, still left in them.

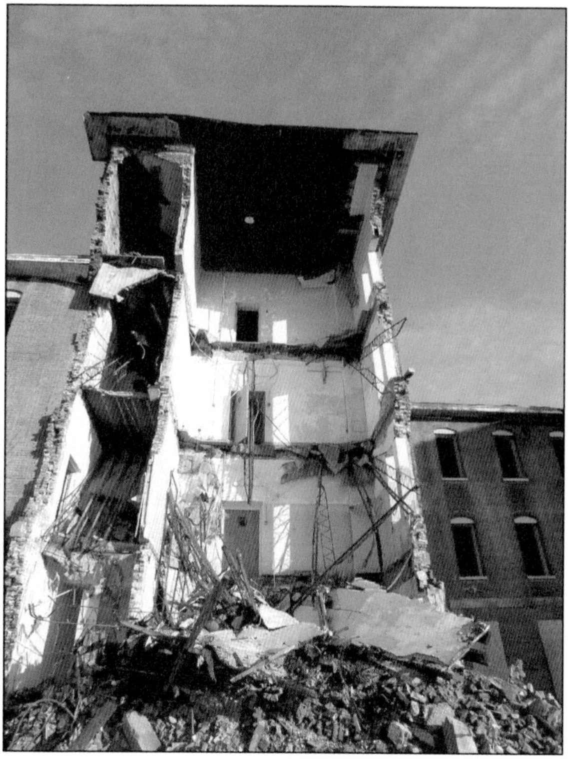

ASC Development wasted no time in demolishing the remaining buildings on the property. This image shows a cross section of Reed Hall. ASC workers poked away at the building with steel beams swung from earthmovers. The end result was a unique revealing of Reed Hall's innards.

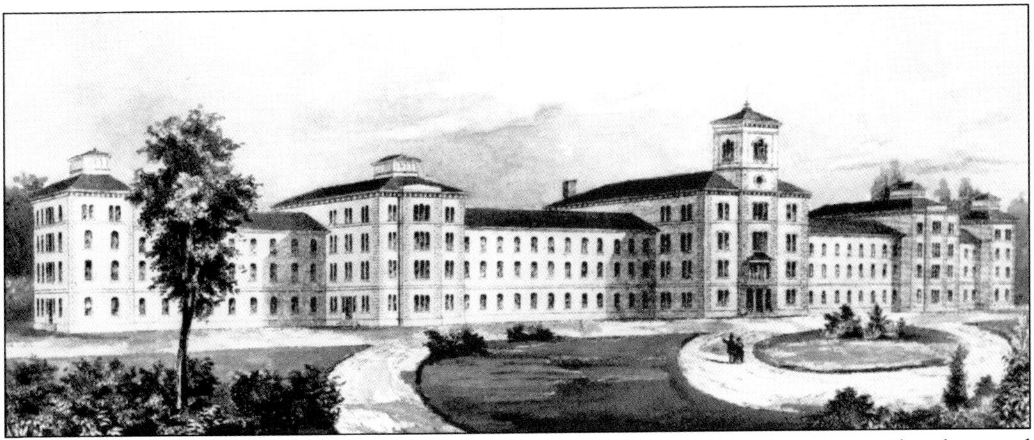

Shown here is the vision of Dixmont from 100 years ago, a stark comparison to the shattered hulk the asylum became. The designs for the retail development that replaced Dixmont—River Pointe Plaza—literally called for a burial of the hospital. The parking lot is designed to be even with the roofline of Reed Hall.

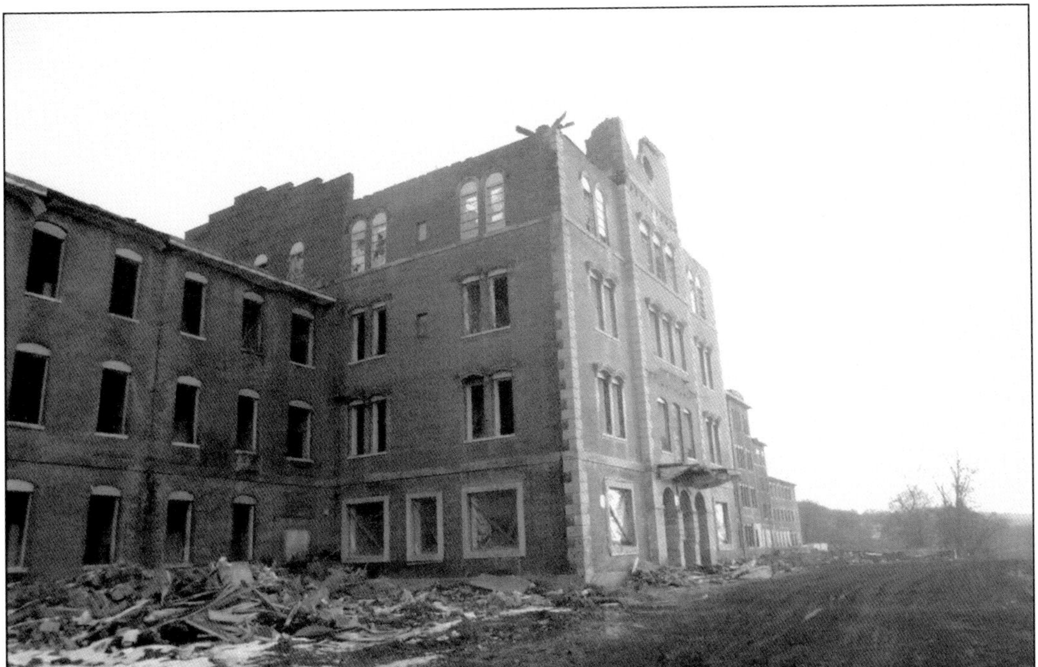

This is a shot of Dixmont in 2004. Despite rumors of closing and budget cuts, Dixmont's administration was seeking to expand its hospital. In addition to serving Beaver and Lawrence Counties, as well as taking in the occasional emergency commitment of Allegheny County residents, officials were devising a way to petition the secretary of public welfare to redesignate Dixmont's service area to include Butler County as well. A 1982–1983 goals and objectives report indicates that a formal proposal was submitted to the central office requesting the redesignation.

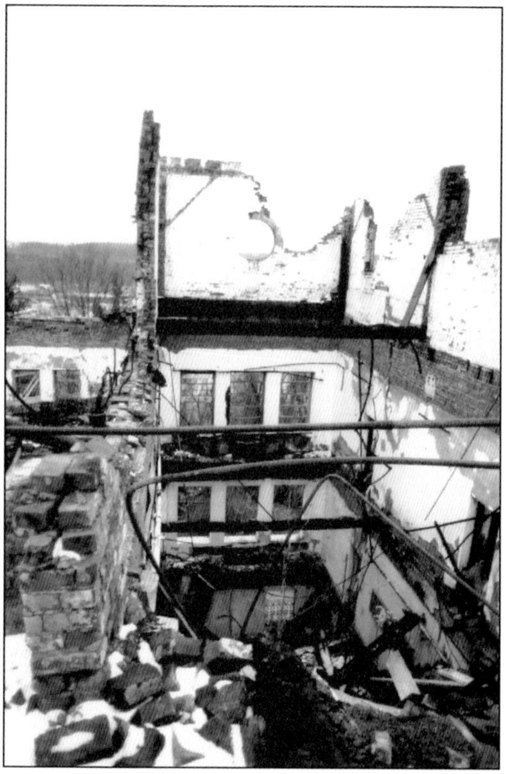

This photograph was taken at the very top of Reed Hall, where the damage of a 1995 fire can clearly be seen. At 10:17 a.m. on Friday, June 2, 1995, smoke was reported to be coming from Dixmont's vicinity. By 10:32 a.m., the first responding fire company arrived. Even though Dixmont was protected by a security company, the company never called to report the fire, nor did they respond to answer the telephone after more than 20 rings.

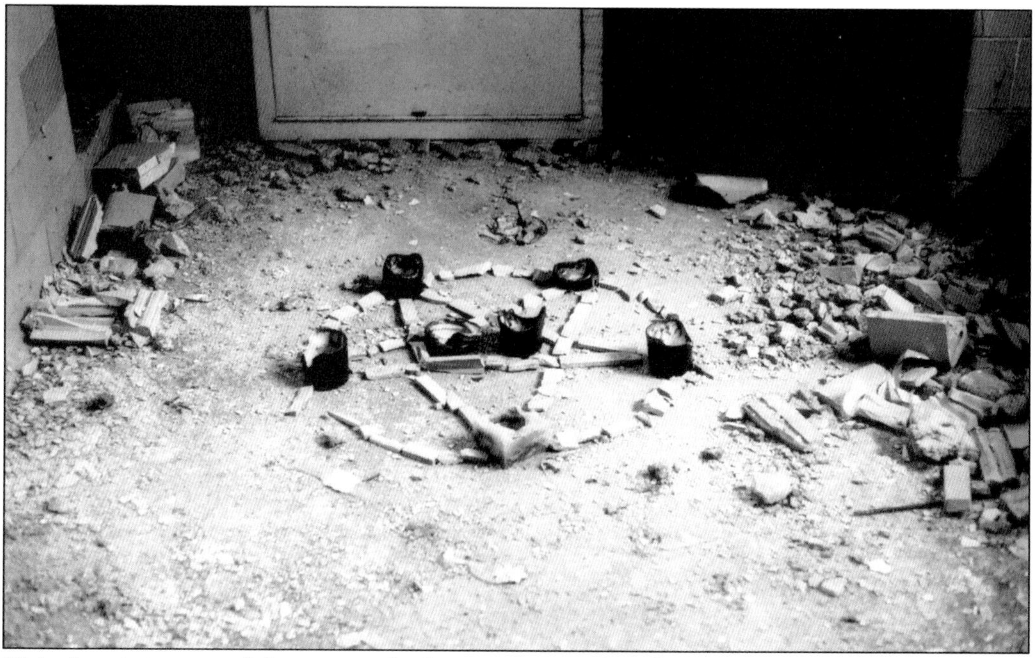

This shot is in one of the patient bathrooms in Reed Hall. On the surface, the pentagram and candles may appear to be part of some satanic ritual. However, amateur filmmakers used Dixmont as a giant set for horror movies. The site was also a backdrop for artistic photography, including nudes.

Patient belongings once occupied these shelves, which still had name tags on them. The goal of Dixmont in its last few years of service was to utilize Reed Hall so that one patient occupied one room. This required acquiring waivers from the state on minimal patient needs. Reed Hall's design did not meet minimum standards, such as minimum cubic feet of living space per room.

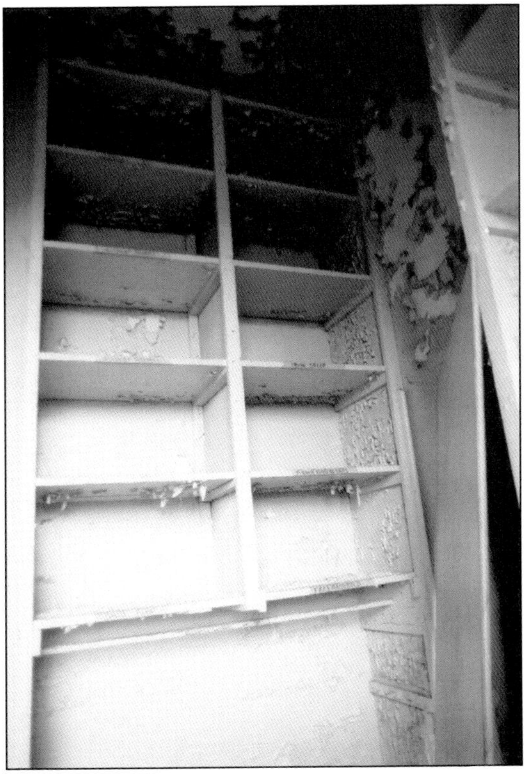

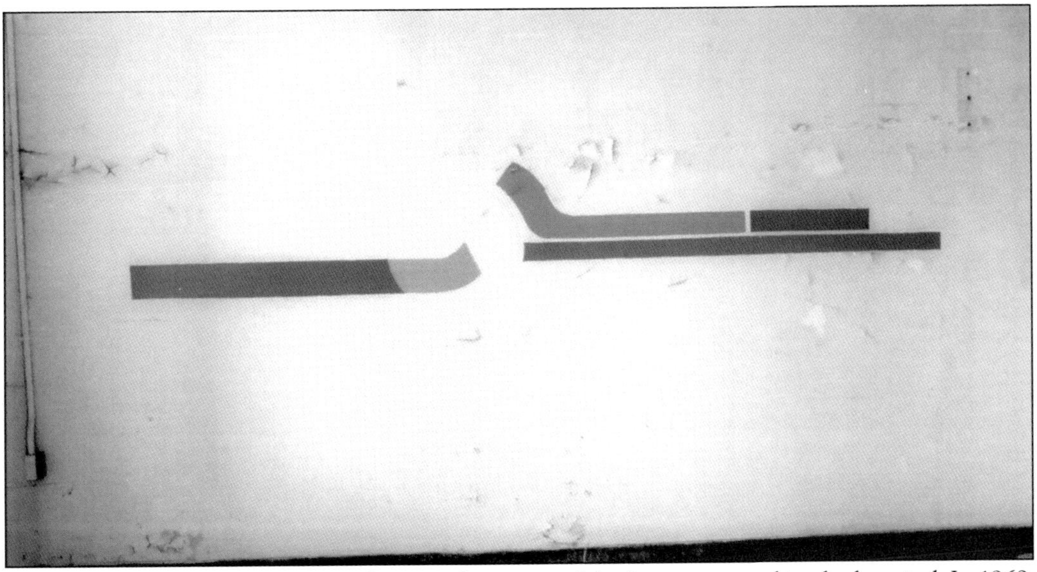

Another example of abstract art, this mural was one of the best preserved in the hospital. In 1969, Dr. Robert Weimer contacted Lawrence T. Good, president of the Architectural Environment Research Foundation in Topeka, Kansas, regarding a complete redesign of Wards A, D, and H in Reed Hall in order to better accommodate patients with a more aesthetic design. The state declined to fund the project. "I think it is terribly shortsighted of the Department to not follow through with this project but as you can well realize I am powerless to do anything about it," Dr. Weimer wrote on July 29, 1969.

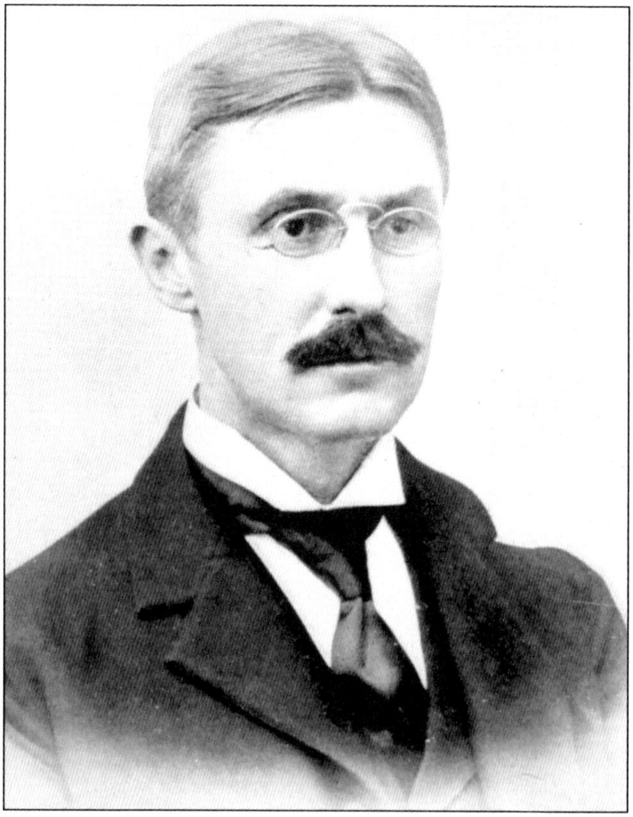

Dr. Henry Hutchinson came to Dixmont as the third assistant physician for the hospital in 1879. Hailing from Trenton, New Jersey, Hutchinson was well received by Dr. Joseph Allison Reed, whose health was precarious at the time. He became Dixmont's second superintendent in November 1884, seven days prior to the death of Dr. Reed. Dr. Hutchinson assumed superintendence over 498 patients, a number that escalated to 538 within his first year. Dr. Hutchinson took an interest in every department of the hospital, striving to continue the work that Dr. Reed started. During his tenure, the board of directors voted to explore the property for placing natural gas wells on the farm in an effort to defray rising energy costs.

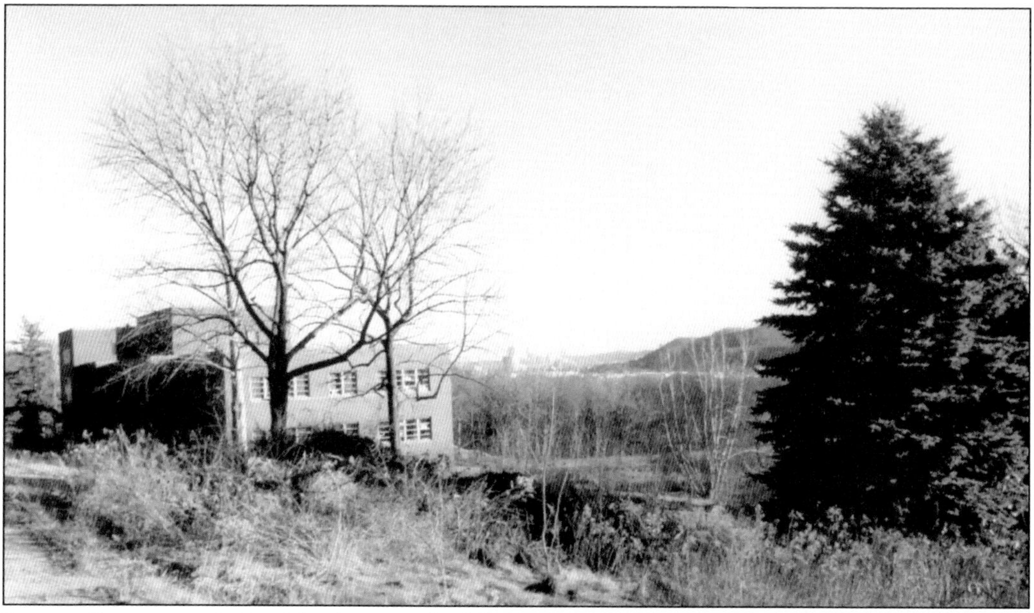

Eventually renamed the Hutchinson Building, the admission and treatment building was dedicated Friday, April 30, 1954. It was named for Dr. Henry Hutchinson, Dixmont's second superintendent. Dr. Hutchinson stepped into his position in 1884, following the death of Dr. Reed. He served for 61 years and died at the age of 92 in 1947. (Courtesy Beth Cummins.)

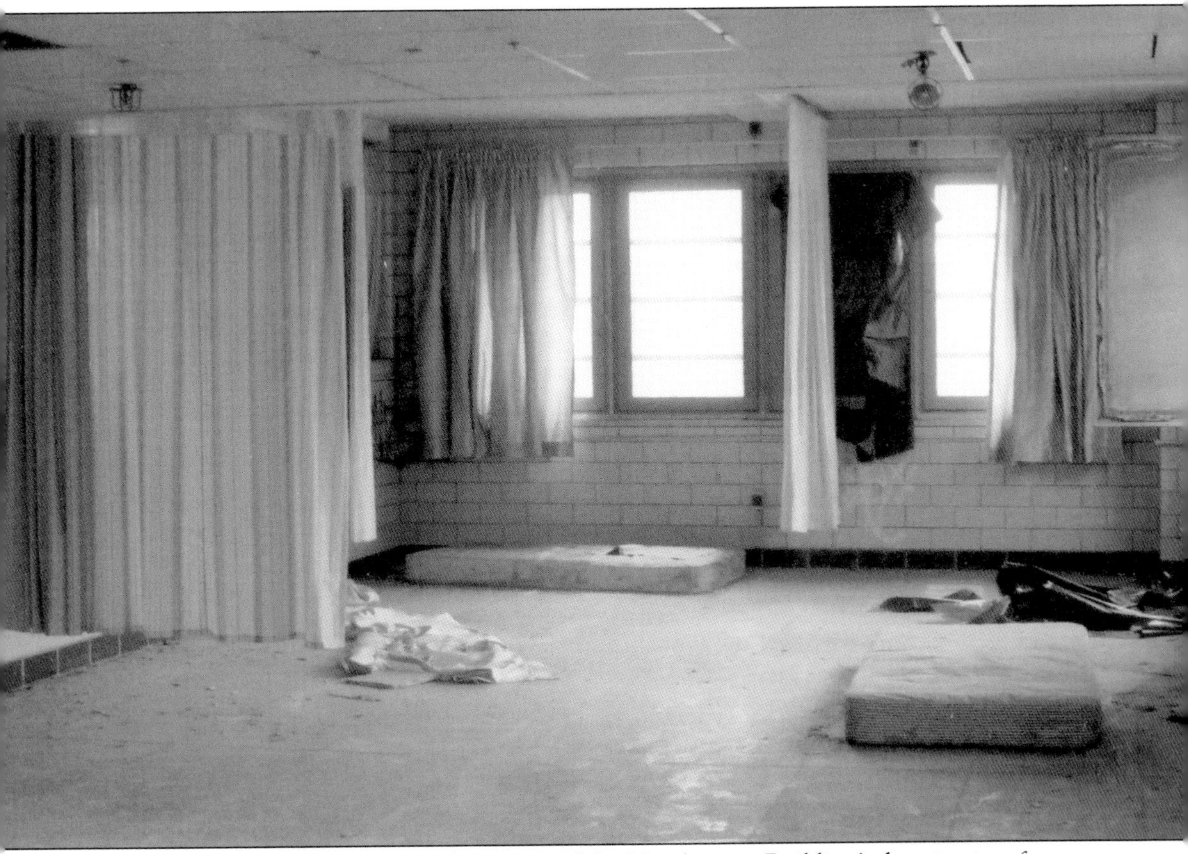

This photograph, taken in 2002, shows one of the Hutchinson Building's dormitories after years of decay. Privacy curtains still separated the beds, and the ceiling tiles are visibly destroyed. The building was described to have a "sterile look that faces you as soon as you walk into the building." The Therapeutic Environment Committee looked into replacing the divider curtains in favor of solid dividers as they did not give sufficient privacy and patients could pull on them and fall.

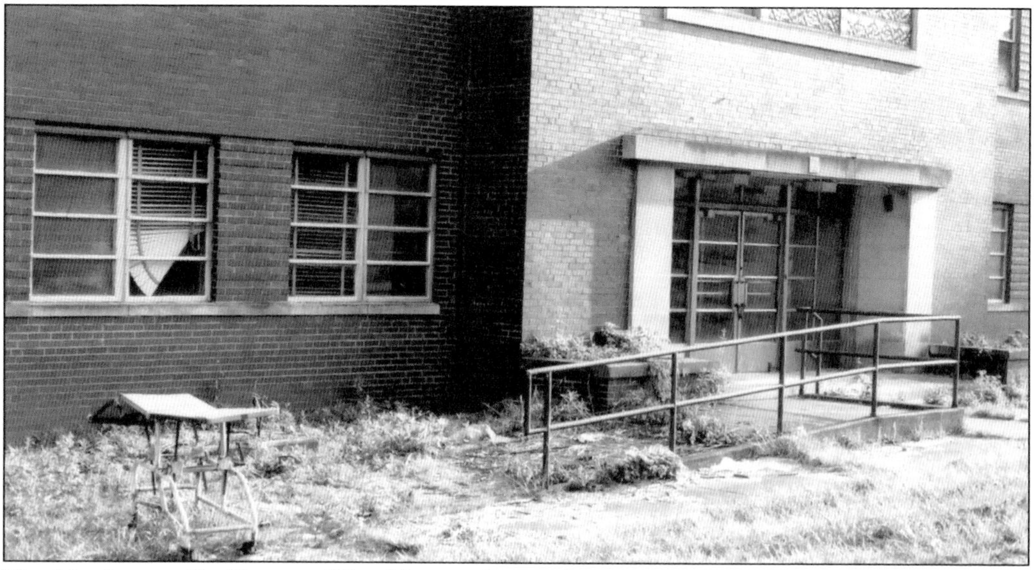

The Hutchinson Building, or "Hutch" to staff, was three stories. The aim at the time of design was "to have the building function as the heart of the institution." The ground floor housed the dining rooms, kitchen, occupational therapy rooms, laboratory, morgue, and X-ray suite. The first floor was for male patients and the second floor for females. Located directly over the first floor lobby and offices was a "small employees infirmary and operating suite for lobotomies and other minor operations."

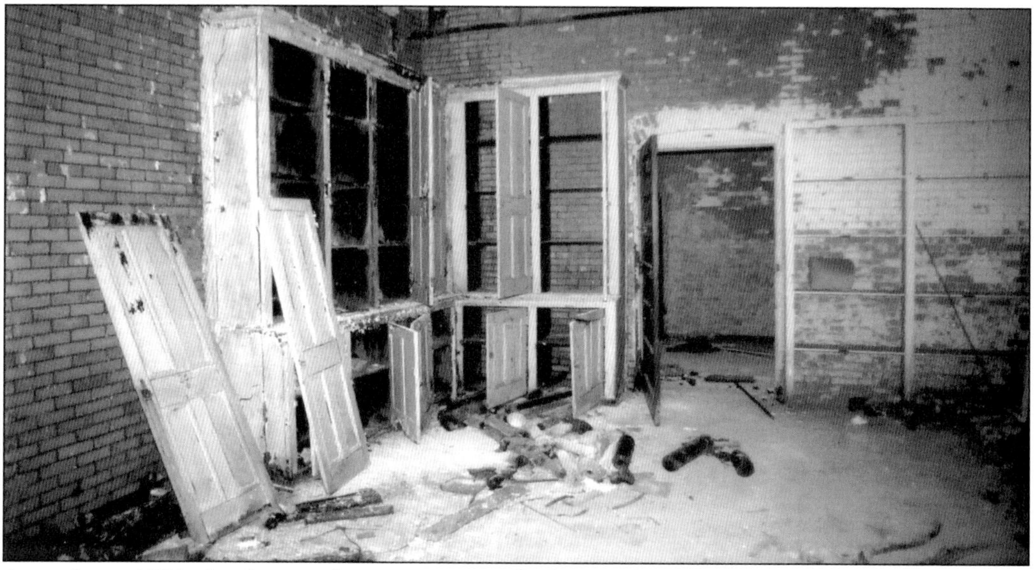

As early as 1974, the dietary department was dealing with issues of organic versus inorganic foods. The January 1974 Dixmont newsletter had an article by a dietary intern that weighed the pros and cons of the argument. Dixmont's food quality ran the spectrum from excellent to abysmal. During the days of Dr. Joseph Allison Reed, the farm provided patients with fresh fruits and vegetables. In the 1940s, *Pittsburgh Post-Gazette* reporter Ray Sprigle wrote an exposé from inside Dixmont, writing that the food was revolting and that meat was missing from most meals. The fare improved by Dr. Robert Weimer's tenure, and, while institutional, Dixmont's food was not remembered as being as bad as Sprigle described.

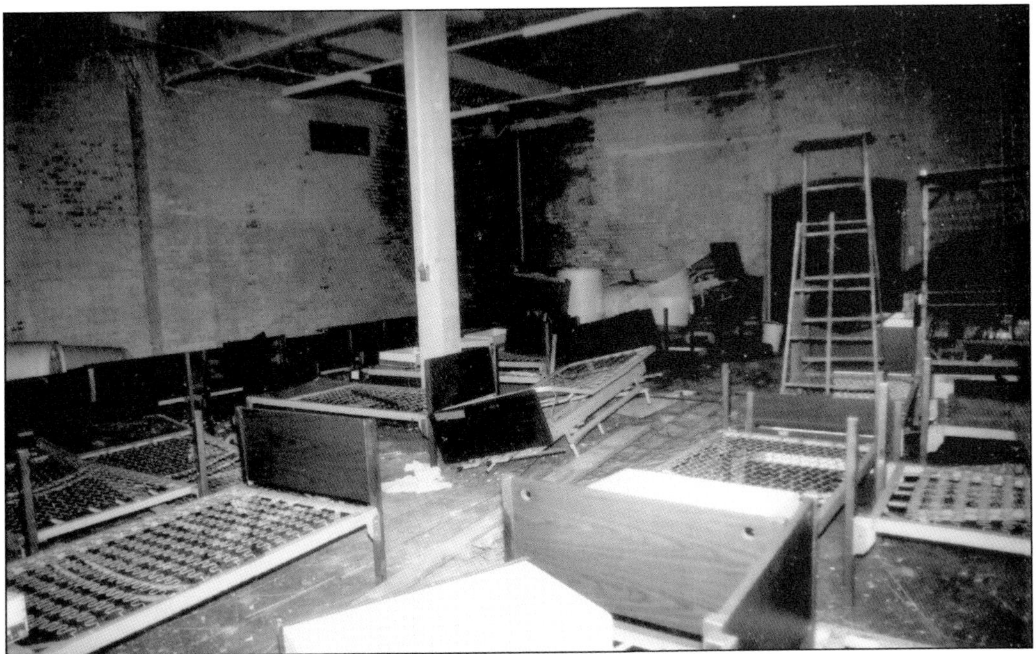

After Dixmont closed, many items were discovered to be left behind. These beds found a new home in the first floor of the dietary building. Not only were the beds left behind, many of them still had patient belongings in their headboard drawers. Tube socks, sticker books, and more were all found.

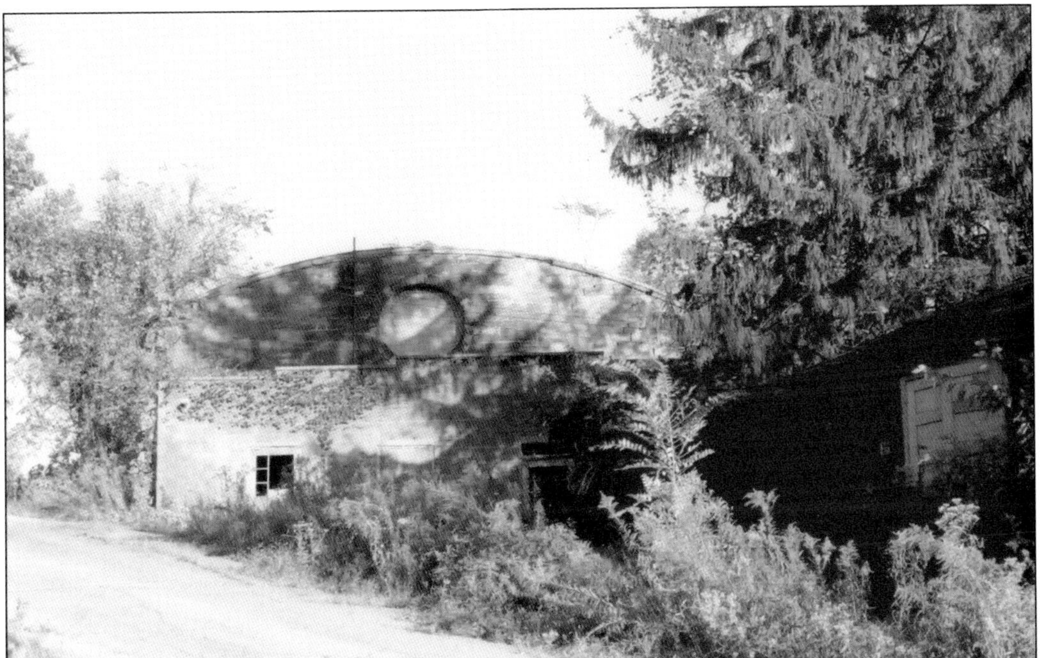

Known as the maintenance building, the original use of this structure was determined to be for washing Dixmont's laundry. It was later converted to a carpenter's shop and maintenance facility. The institution's laundry eventually got its own building.

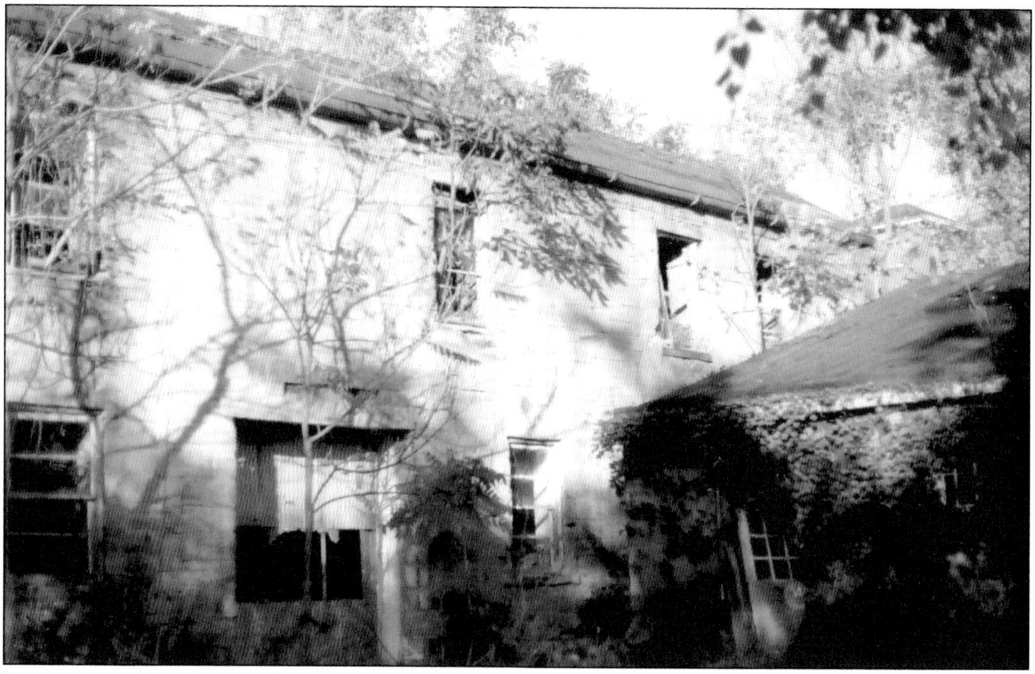

In more modern times, the maintenance department, headed by Kenneth R. Viney, included carpenters, electricians, mechanics, drivers, painters, and plumbers. The team ensured that all of Dixmont kept running efficiently. The scope of the department included all buildings and grounds and maintaining the hospital's water and sewage plants.

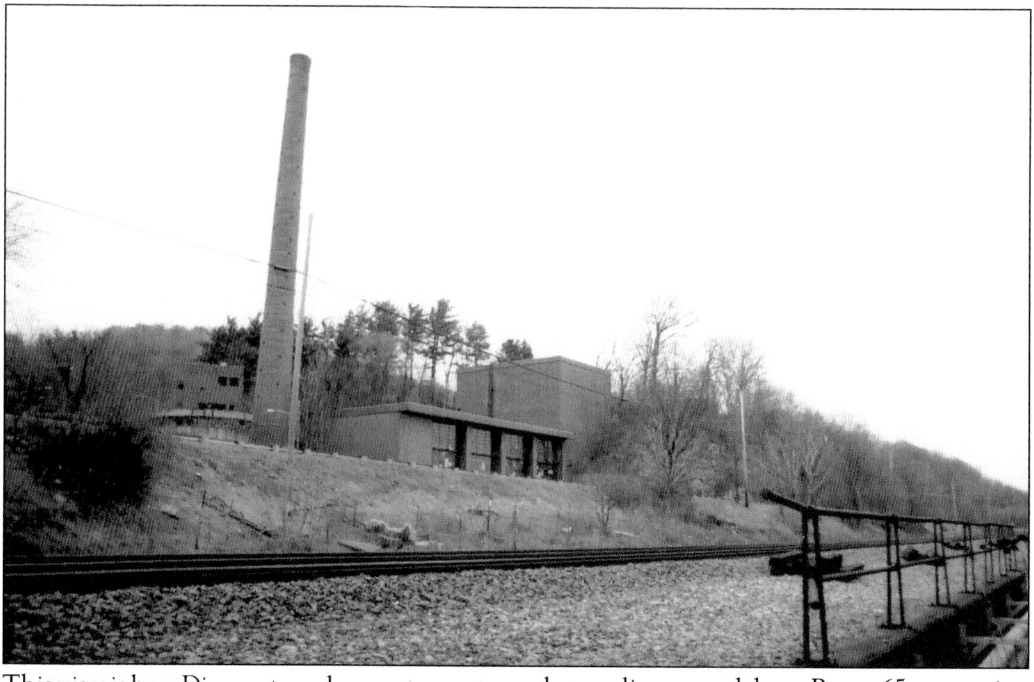

This view is how Dixmont was known to most people traveling up and down Route 65, a towering smokestack attached to an abandoned boiler house. Having been a coal-burning facility, the boiler house was cited for air pollution in 1970. Plans to convert the fuel source to oil followed.

Five

Demolition

On March 7, 2002, Tony Chammas of ASC Development unveiled plans for a large-scale retail development on the site of Dixmont State Hospital. While Kilbuck Township supervisors were eager to get the site back on the tax rolls, the public was not convinced that a retail development would be ideal for the site. On Tuesday, April 16, 2002, the project received conditional approval from the Kilbuck Township supervisors.

While residents stormed this and subsequent meetings to try and block the development, prior meetings for a 400-unit residential development were sparsely attended. In fact, the Stroyne family entertained many potential developers for the site. The stumbling block was finding a developer with deep enough pockets to remediate more than $1 million worth of asbestos in the buildings. Rumors of deeper contamination of the site ran rampant, but an environmental study showed that the site had no more contamination than one would expect from 100 years of vibrant hospital life. The soil beneath the garage had some petroleum by-products, but nothing that would threaten a water supply. Rumors of buried medical waste or toxic materials were dispelled. The project garnered support from Neville and Ohio Townships and Avalon Borough officials, who passed resolutions in favor of the development.

ASC had a budget of $28 million to work with. The projected was expected to generate about $300,000 in taxes for the township and school district. The plan passed the planning commission by a five-to-one vote. Early December saw the implosion of Dixmont's boiler house smokestack, but tearing down Reed Hall would not be so neat. Backhoes equipped with giant claws grabbed swung steel beams as though they were chopsticks and poked them into Reed Hall's brickwork. The work began on the Lawrence side of the building and moved eastward toward the Beaver units. The job was estimated to take about two weeks but wound up being over a month that spanned the Christmas and New Year holidays.

By the end of 2005, Dixmont's developers had secured the necessary permits to begin their demolition. Wasting no time, larger earthmovers that sat dormant on the site for nearly a year rolled up the disintegrating driveways to make way for progress.

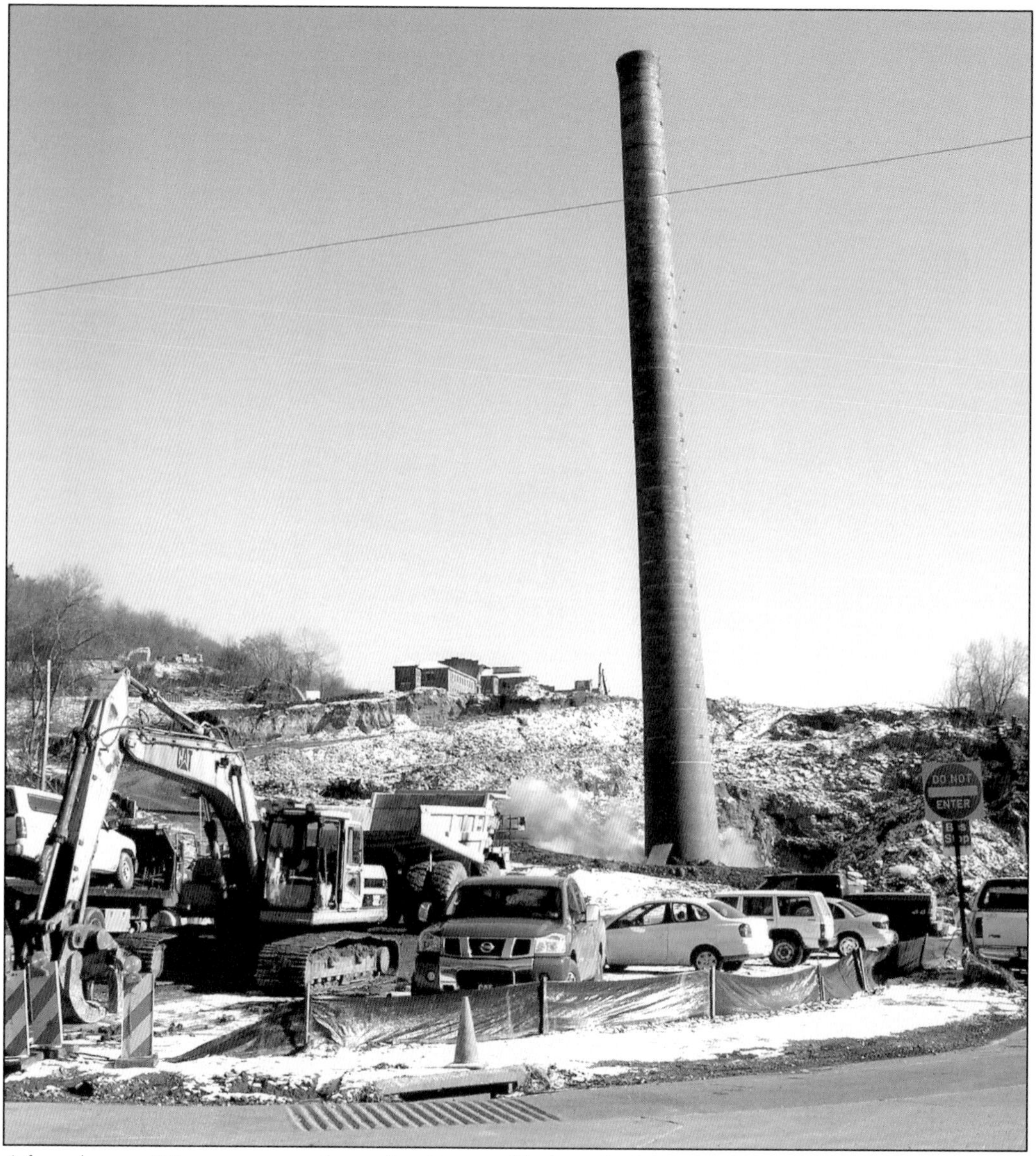

After closure, Dixmont went through a litany of bids to find a buyer. One of the first bids on the property was for $2.7 million from Kilbuck Associates, which planned on developing the site for a Ross Township company named Med-Chek Laboratories. The company planned to base Med-Chek's headquarters on the property, as well as develop an 18-hole golf course and a residential component of mixed single and multifamily housing. Kilbuck Associates contested the sale of the property, however, claiming the state did not disclose buried wells and pollutants on the site. They filed a lawsuit, which was withdrawn after years of appeals.

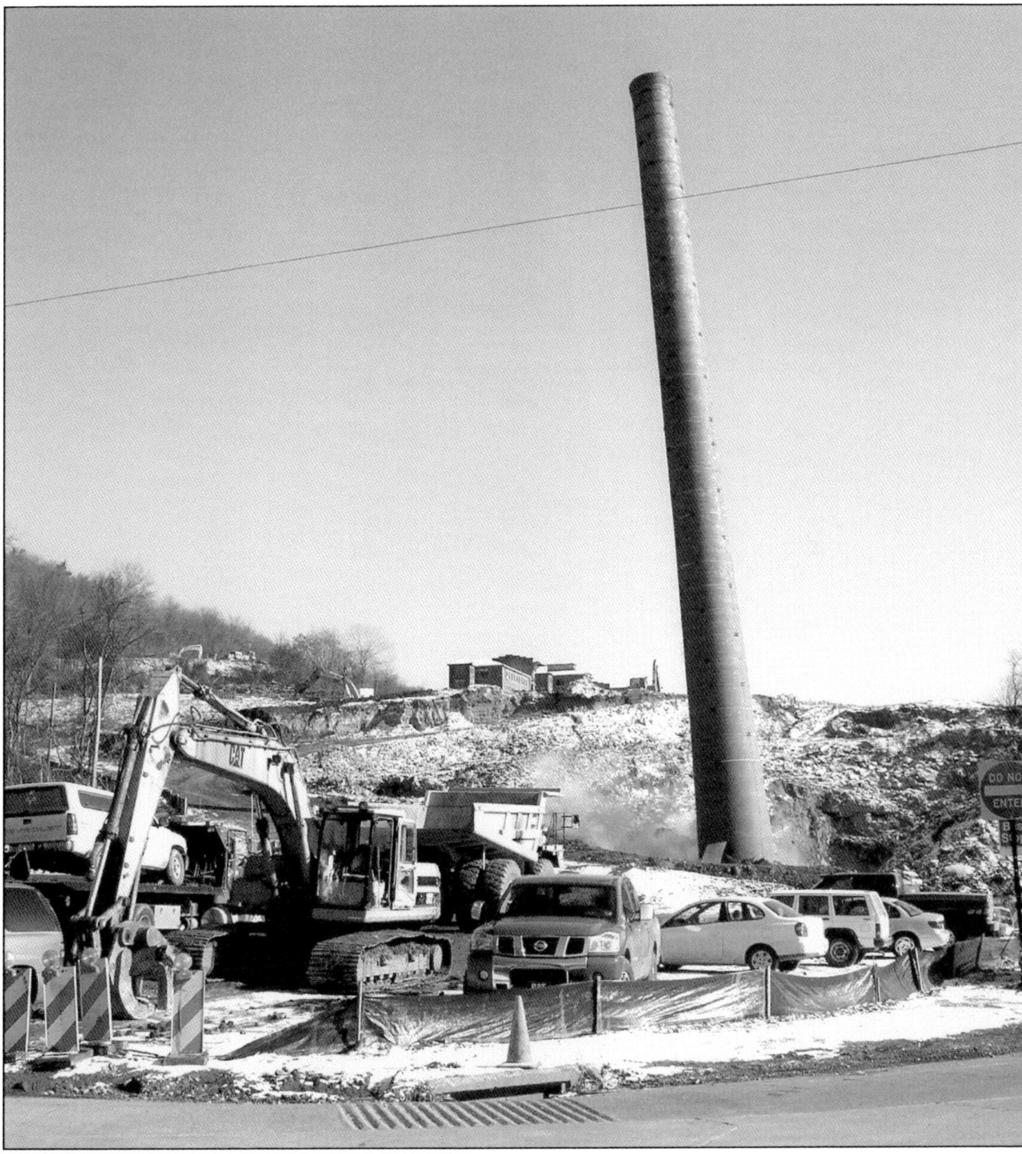

The Dixmont property was appraised at $5.08 million in 1986. By 1989, a reappraisal dropped that figure to $2.3 million. After the Stroyne family purchased the property in 1999, the Allegheny County Board of Property Assessment mistakenly assessed the value of the property at $15 million—the value of the property if it were a functioning hospital. Ralph Stroyne appealed and the assessment was lowered to $1.5 million. Stroyne tried to make money off his investment by selling off parcels of the property and harvesting the trees. He also sold the scrap metal from the buildings and optioned portions of the property off to potential developers.

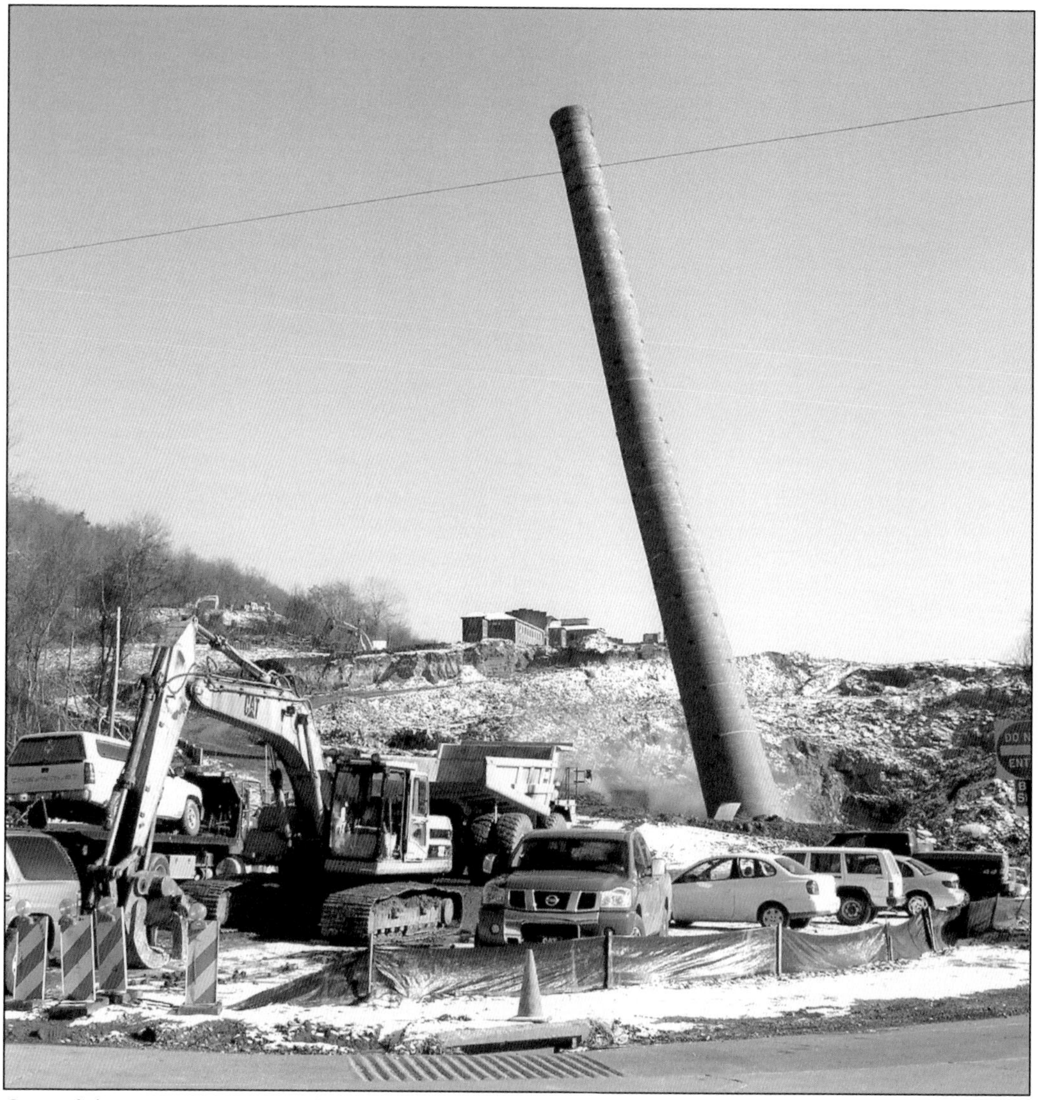

One of the more promising plans for the site was put on the table shortly before Dixmont even closed. State representative David Mayernik proposed a bill that would have sold 188 acres and their buildings to St. John's Hospital for $1. The deadline for the proposition coincided with the deadline for the state budget—June 30—despite being approved by the appropriations and rules committees the very same day it was introduced. The legislature failed to come to a consensus on the proposal and it subsequently died, forcing the sale of the hospital into the standard general services bidding process for surplus properties. A sale to St. John's was estimated to provide as many as 300 new jobs. Plans called for installing nearly 200 beds in the Cammarata and Hutchinson Buildings.

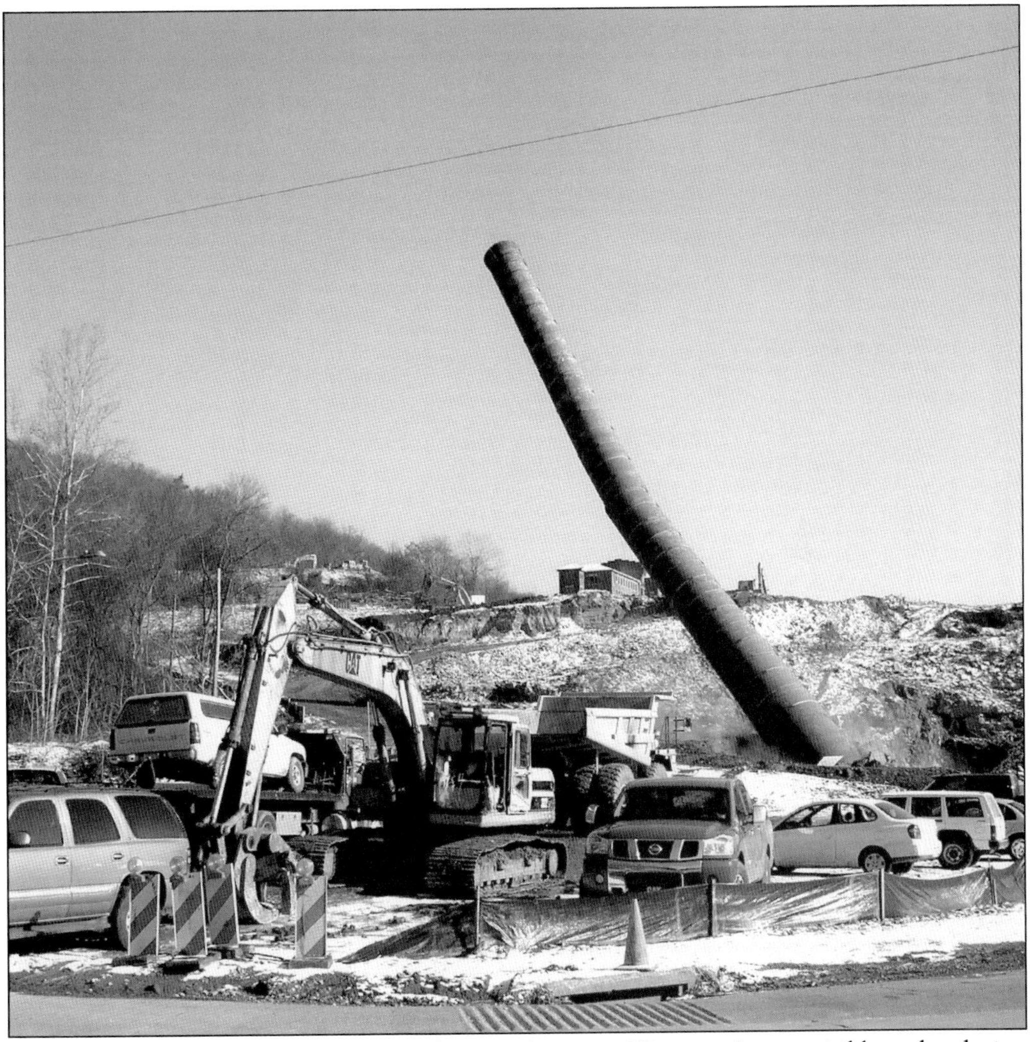

The demolition of the smokestack brought an end to one of Dixmont's most visible and enduring landmarks. Demolition experts carefully prepared the smokestack so that it would not fall across Route 65. The implosion was flawless and the giant chimney gracefully fell backward onto Dixmont's Tom's Run entrance driveway.

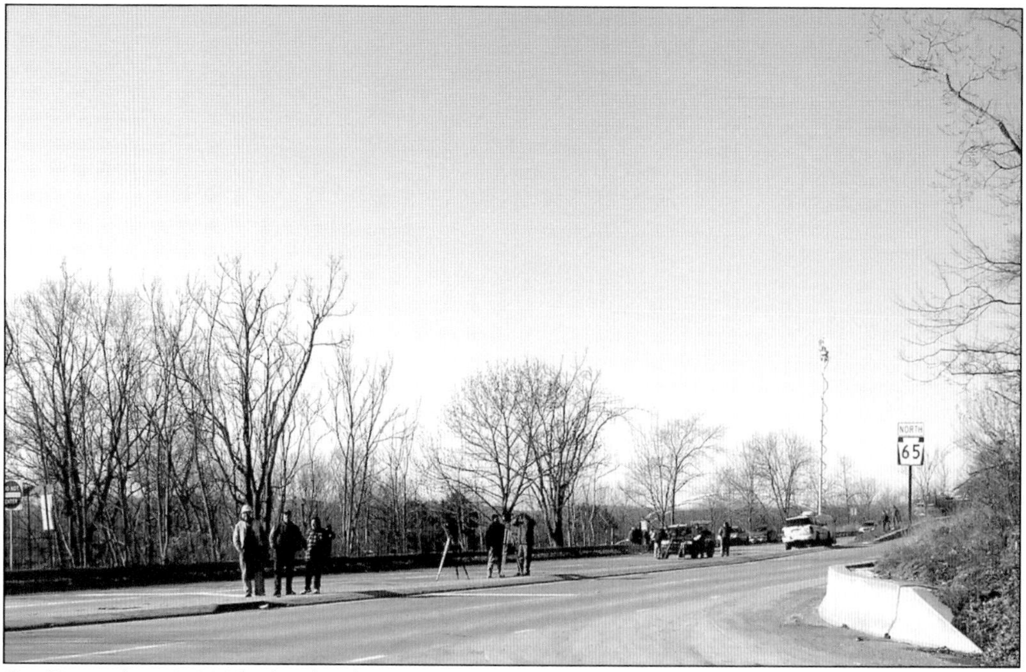

On December 6, 2005, the developers and the media gathered to watch the implosion of the most visible part of Dixmont—the boiler house smokestack along Route 65. Originally slated for a 10:30 a.m. implosion, the stack fell shortly before noon, while police stopped traffic in both directions for safety.

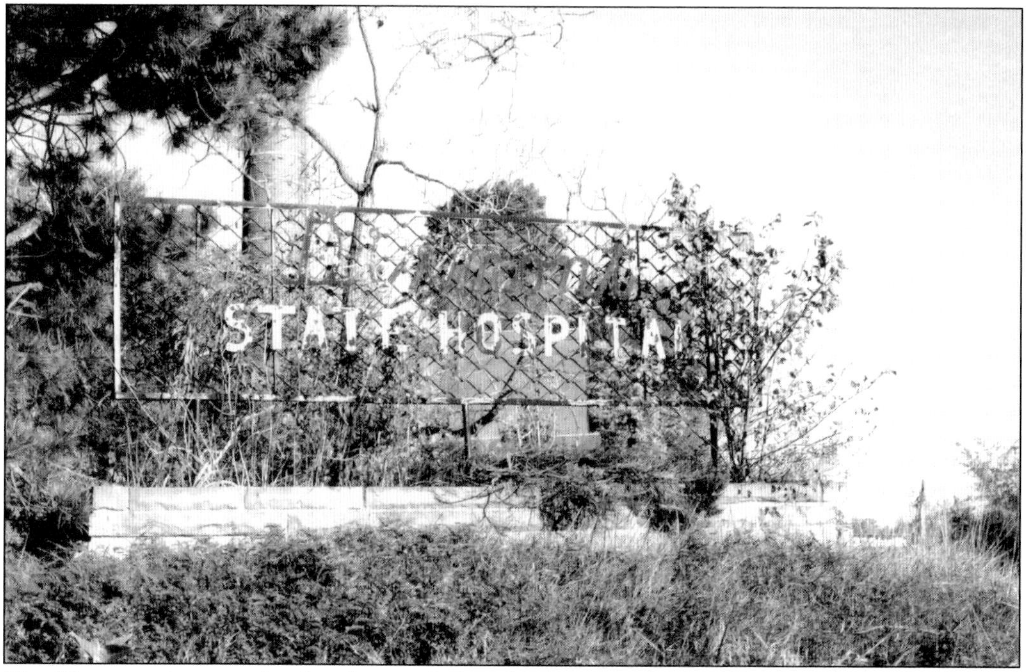

The Dixmont sign, another familiar symbol to those passing by on Route 65, stood on a knoll at the foot of the boiler house. It was removed several years prior to the demolition and now finds shelter in the garage of a member of the Ben Avon Area Historical Association.

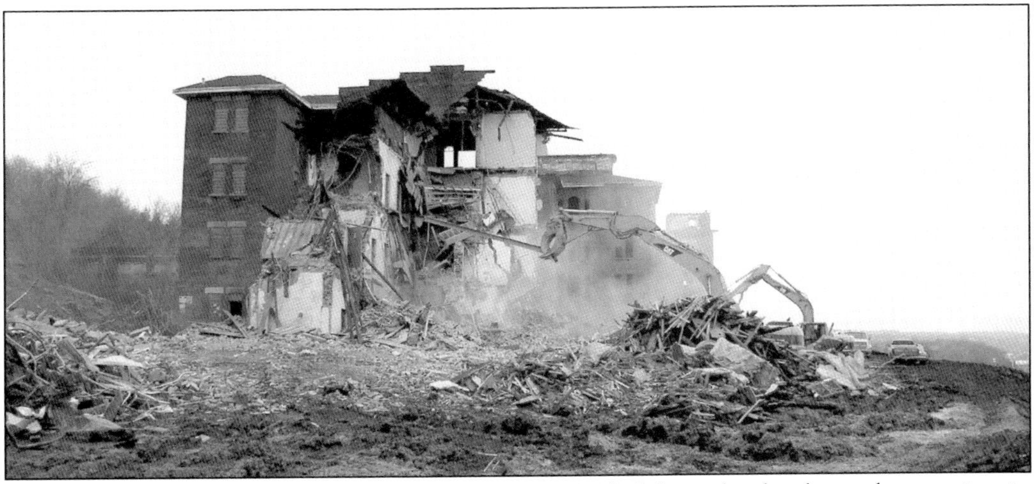

Working over the Christmas and New Year 2005–2006 holidays, the developers lost no time in moving forward with the demolition of Reed Hall. It took several weeks to complete this phase of the project. The team of backhoes used loose beams and other large pieces of rubble to skewer the walls of Reed Hall, bringing it to the ground almost effortlessly.

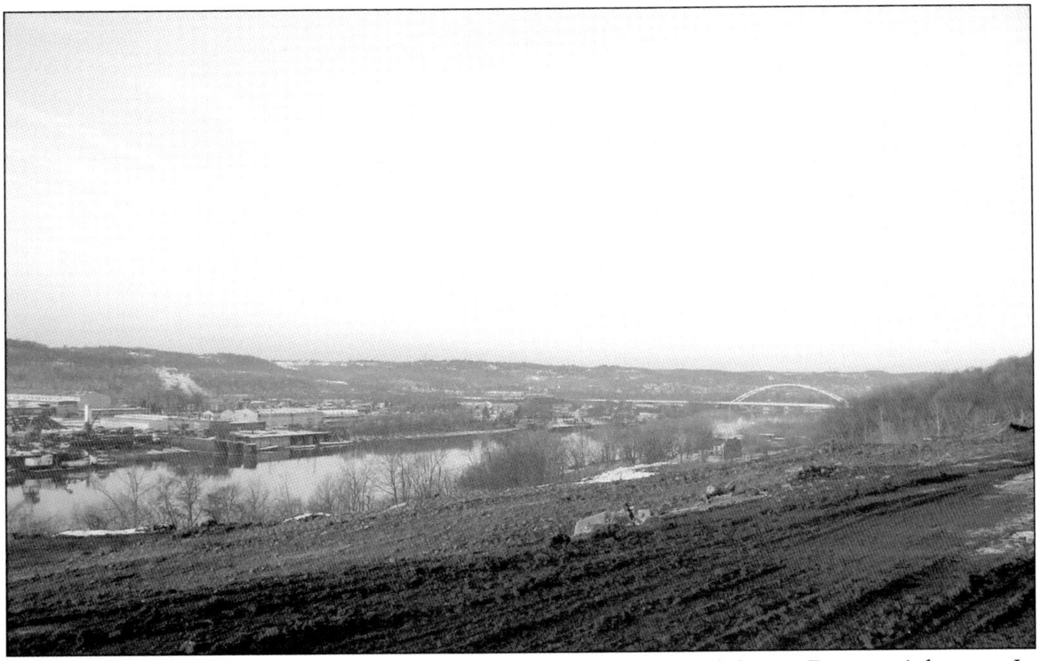

This present-day view of Neville Island shows how much changed during Dixmont's history. In the background is the Interstate 79 bridge, which carries one of the main north-south interstates in western Pennsylvania. The interchange alleviated much of the traffic along Route 65 and allowed better access to Dixmont. Neville Island is still the home of industrial plants and some residential properties.

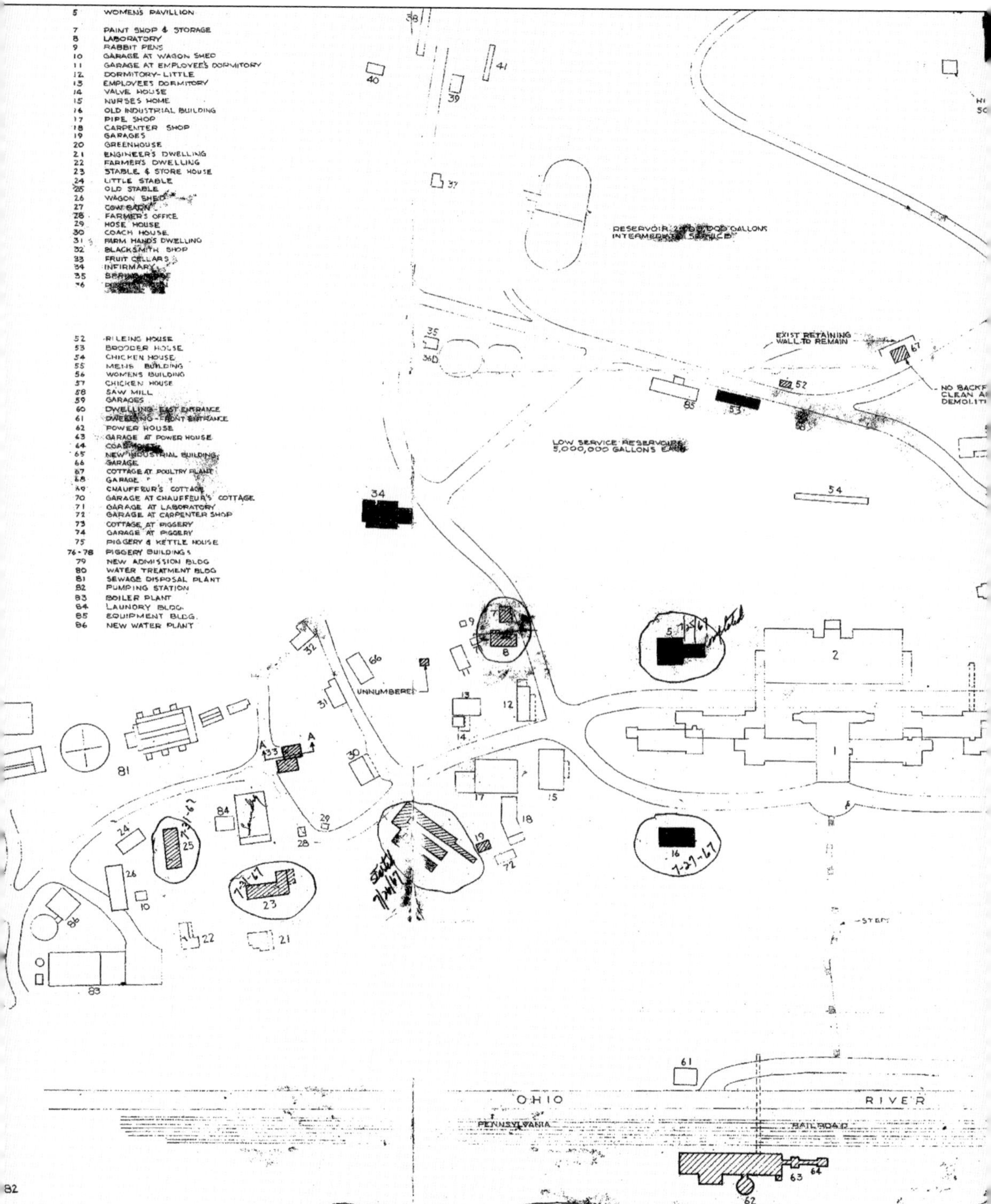

This map was used in the historic remediation of the site. On it, more than 80 different structures appear. Christine Davis Consultants were retained by ASC Development to perform an archeological site survey of Dixmont. Her report verified the accurate locations of the various

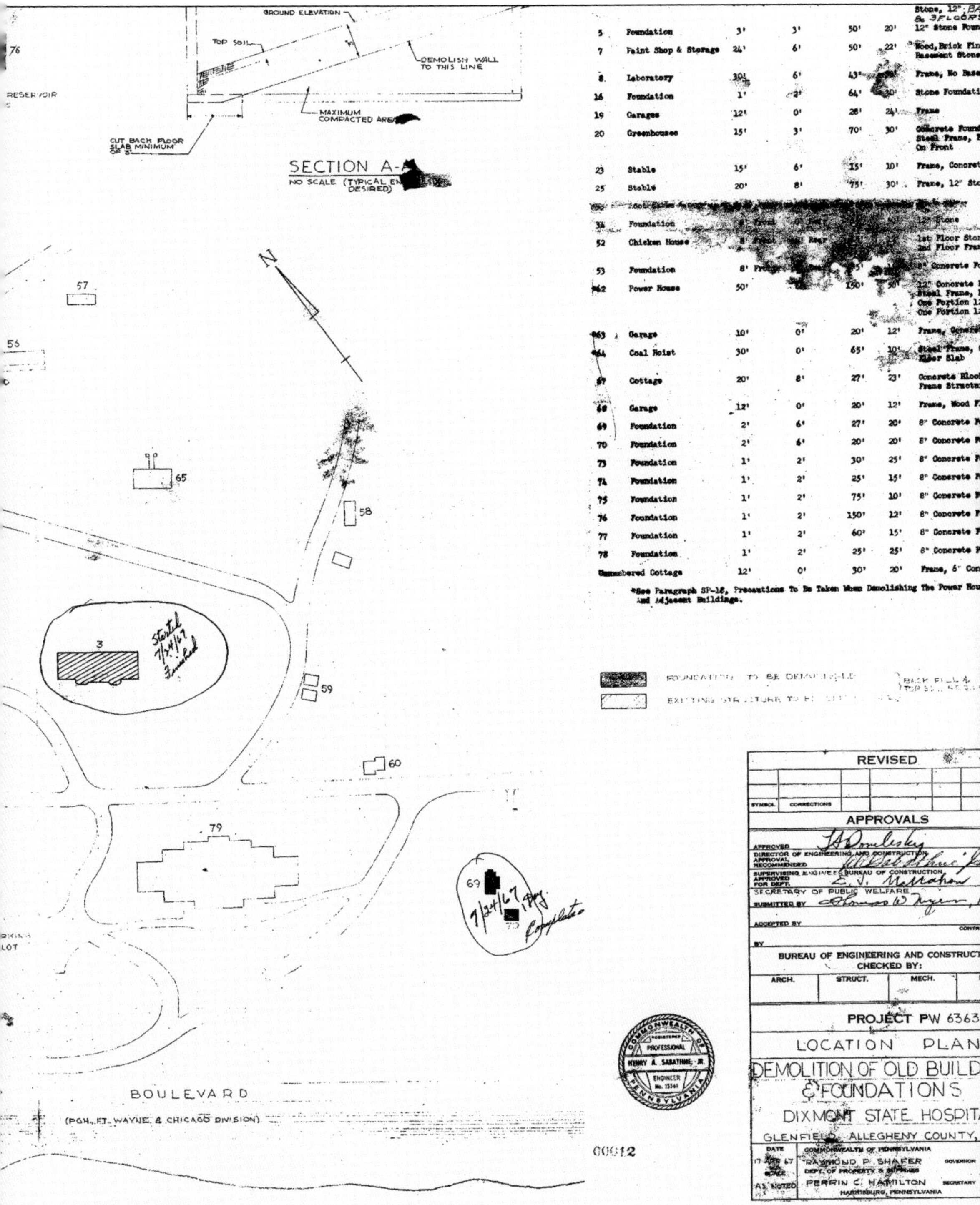

buildings. Because Reed Hall was a national historic landmark, the property had to be preserved through pictures and narrative for future generations.

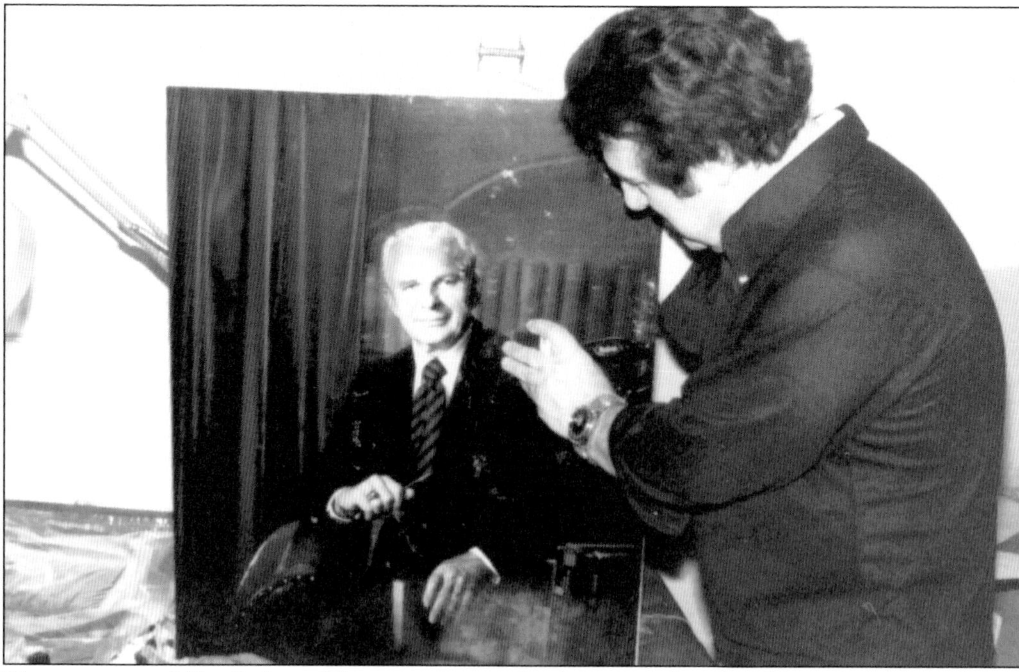

The portrait of Dr. Robert Weimer receives finishing touches by the artist. A portrait of Dr. Joseph Allison Reed was presented to Dixmont in 1886 by his son, James. That portrait hung in the main office of Dixmont and was later moved to the entrance of Reed Hall.

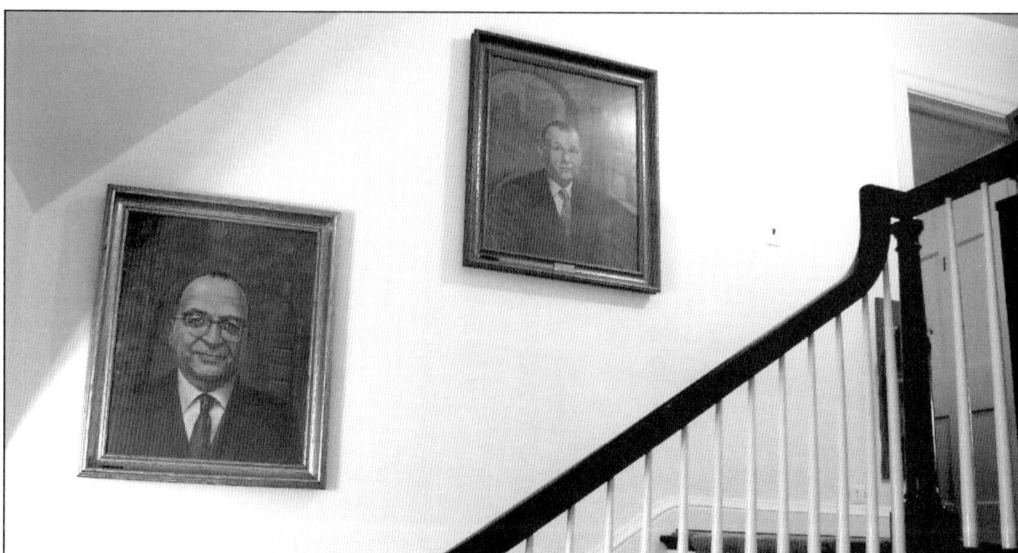

The portraits of past superintendents hang in the Mary T. Summers Volunteer Center at Mayview State Hospital. Here the portraits of Dr. Joseph Cammarata and Dr. Karl Ludwig hang in a stairwell, seen by a select few. There were six superintendents during Dixmont's life, Dr. Joseph Allison Reed, Dr. Henry Hutchinson, Dr. Leonard Rosenzweig, Dr. Joseph Cammarata, Dr. Robert Weimer, and Dr. Karl Ludwig, who assumed superintendence on February 25, 1980. He would quit 16 months later, leaving the hospital in the hands of acting superintendent, Dr. T. E. Thompson.

Dr. Henry Hutchinson's portrait hangs at Mayview State Hospital as well. Dr. Hutchinson's tenure was so long, he became Superintendent Emeritus of Dixmont. He died at the age of 97.

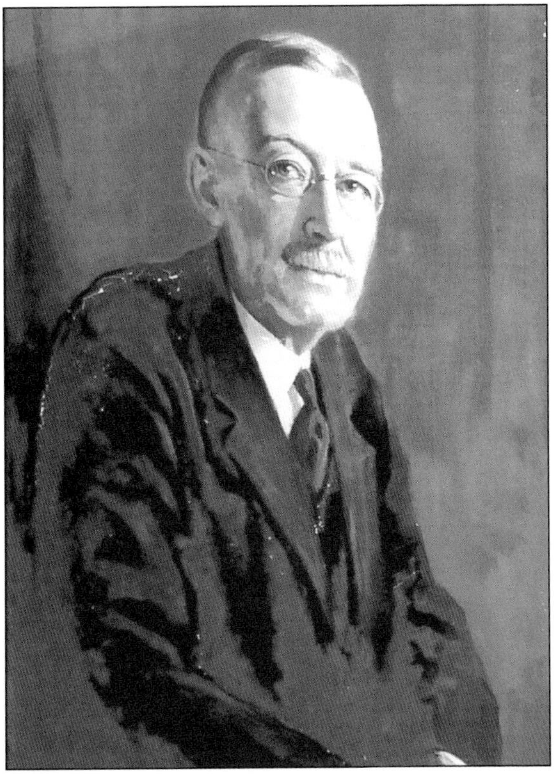

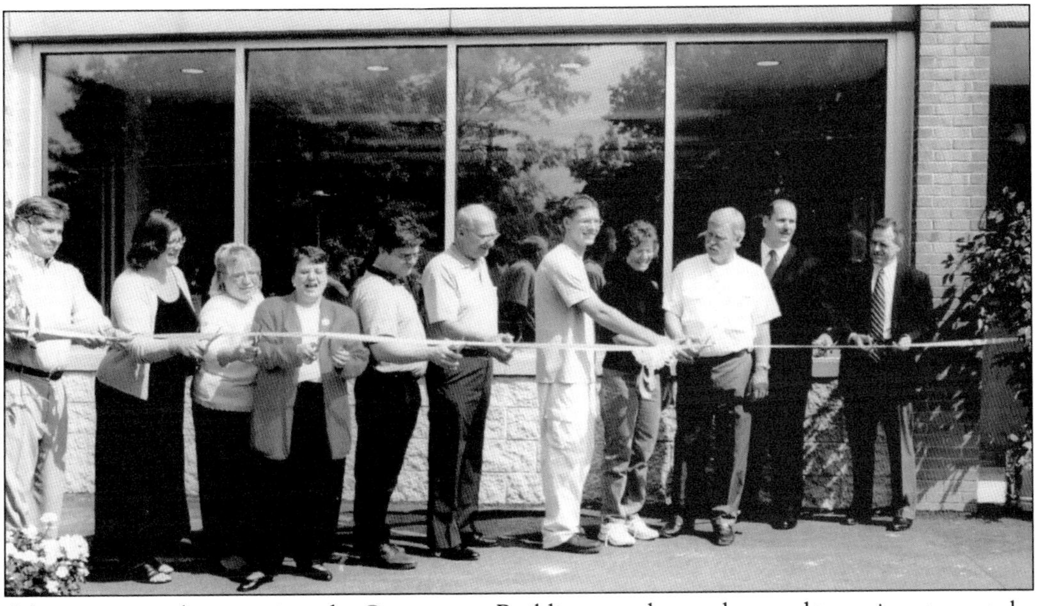

After repairs and renovation, the Cammarata Building was shopped around to various tenants by the Stroyne family. One potential tenant, a $3.4 million drug rehabilitation clinic, drew public outcry. Ralph Stroyne turned down the offer and the money to seek other clients to appease the neighborhood. Part of the building is now home to the Verland Foundation. The other part is home to the Glen Montessori School. Shown here is the 2001 ribbon-cutting celebration for the school's opening in its new location. (Courtesy Connie Rankin/the Citizen.)

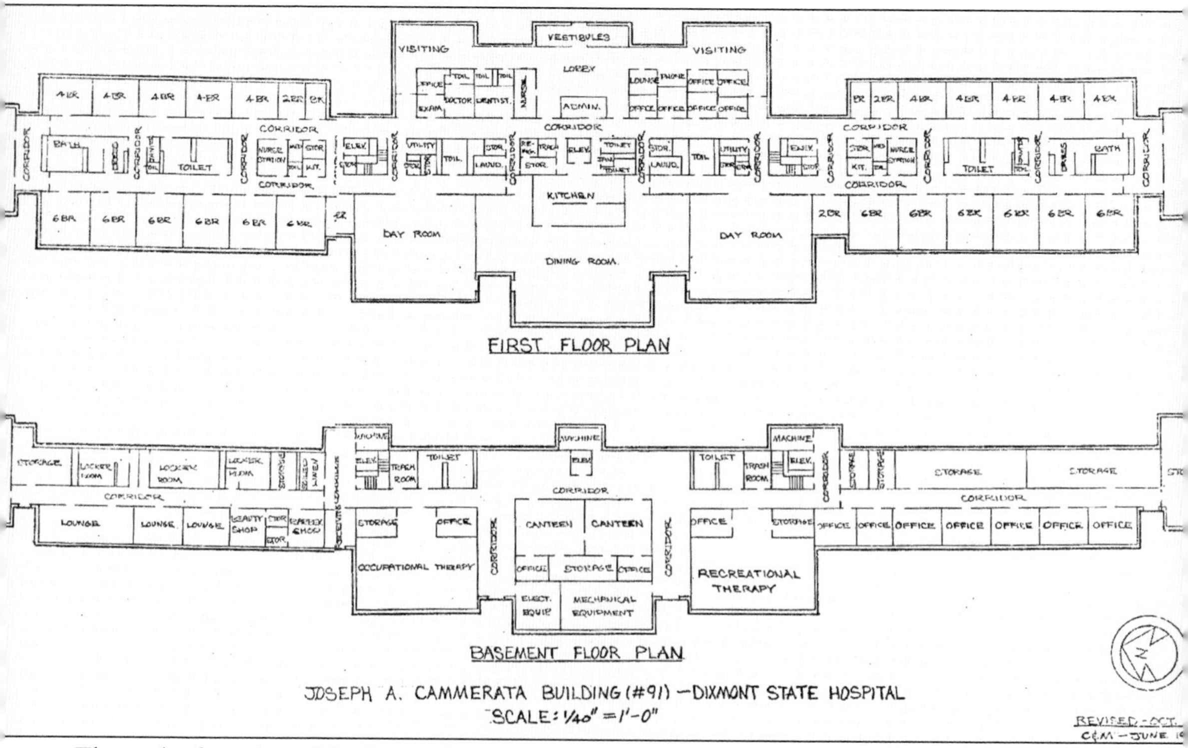

This is the floor plan of the former Cammarata Building. The building's psychiatrist was Dr. Robert Wittig, and Dr. Anibal Herrera was physician. There were four wards in the unit, referred to as "teams." Each team had four to eight patients that were seeking independence and eventual placement back into the community. The teams took many off-site trips to immerse themselves in the community and regain rudimentary skills, such as comparison-shopping, money management, and proper social behavior. The teams met every morning from 9 to 10 in a group therapy session that focused on behavior modification. A report written by Beryl Johnson stated that the activities included "simple self care skills" such as brushing teeth, making telephone calls, and learning to use automatic laundry machines. The teams used the Dixmont bus to take off-site day trips to Pittsburgh or the surrounding county parks.

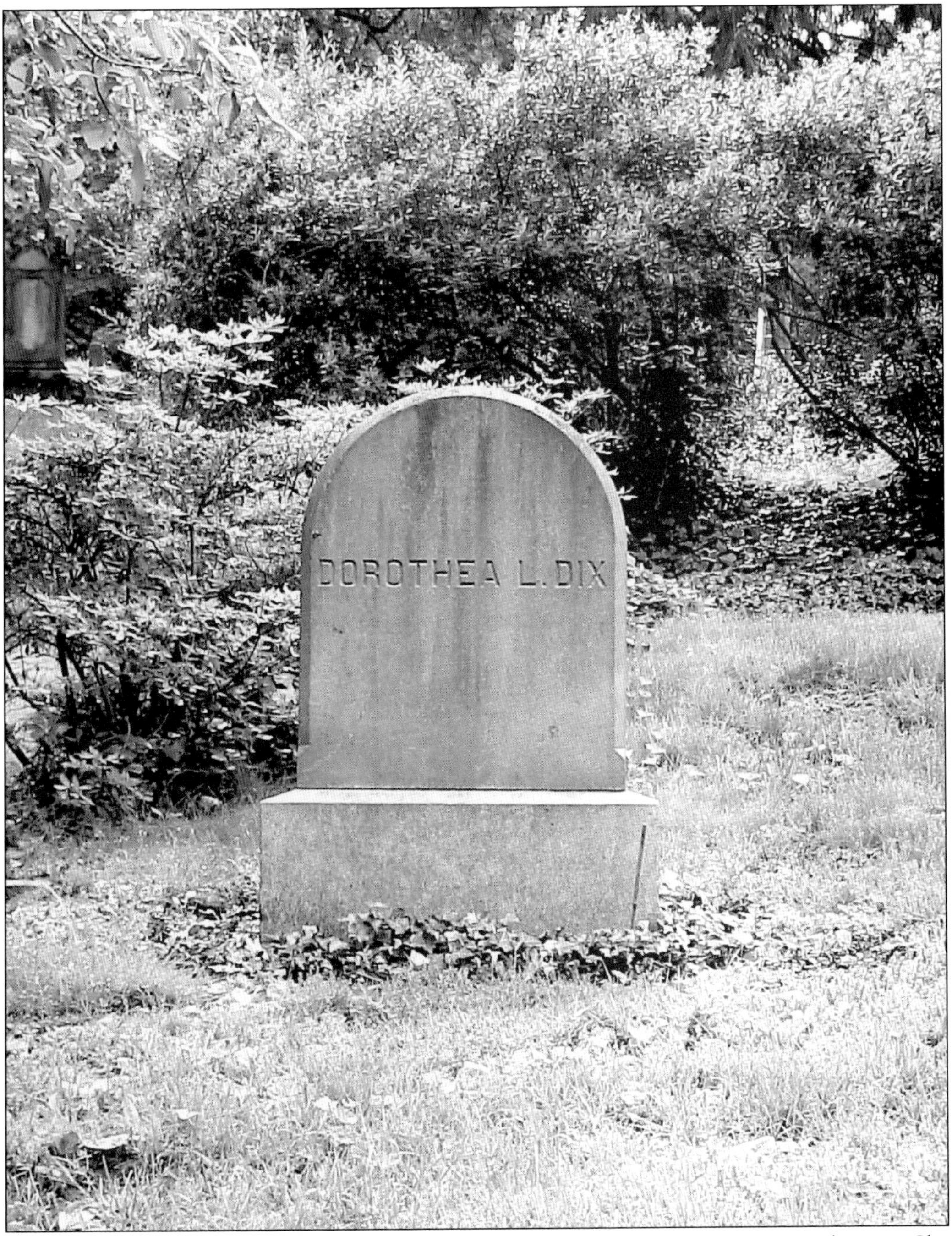

Dorothea Lynde Dix's grave is in Mount Auburn Cemetery in Cambridge, Massachusetts. She died in on July 17, 1887, at her private apartment in the New Jersey State Hospital. Her role as a mental health care reformer took her to the heights of notoriety in her day, so much so that her gravestone has no dates for her birth and death. It was assumed that history would never forget the woman who changed so much for so many. (Courtesy Anna Schuleit and www.1856.org.)

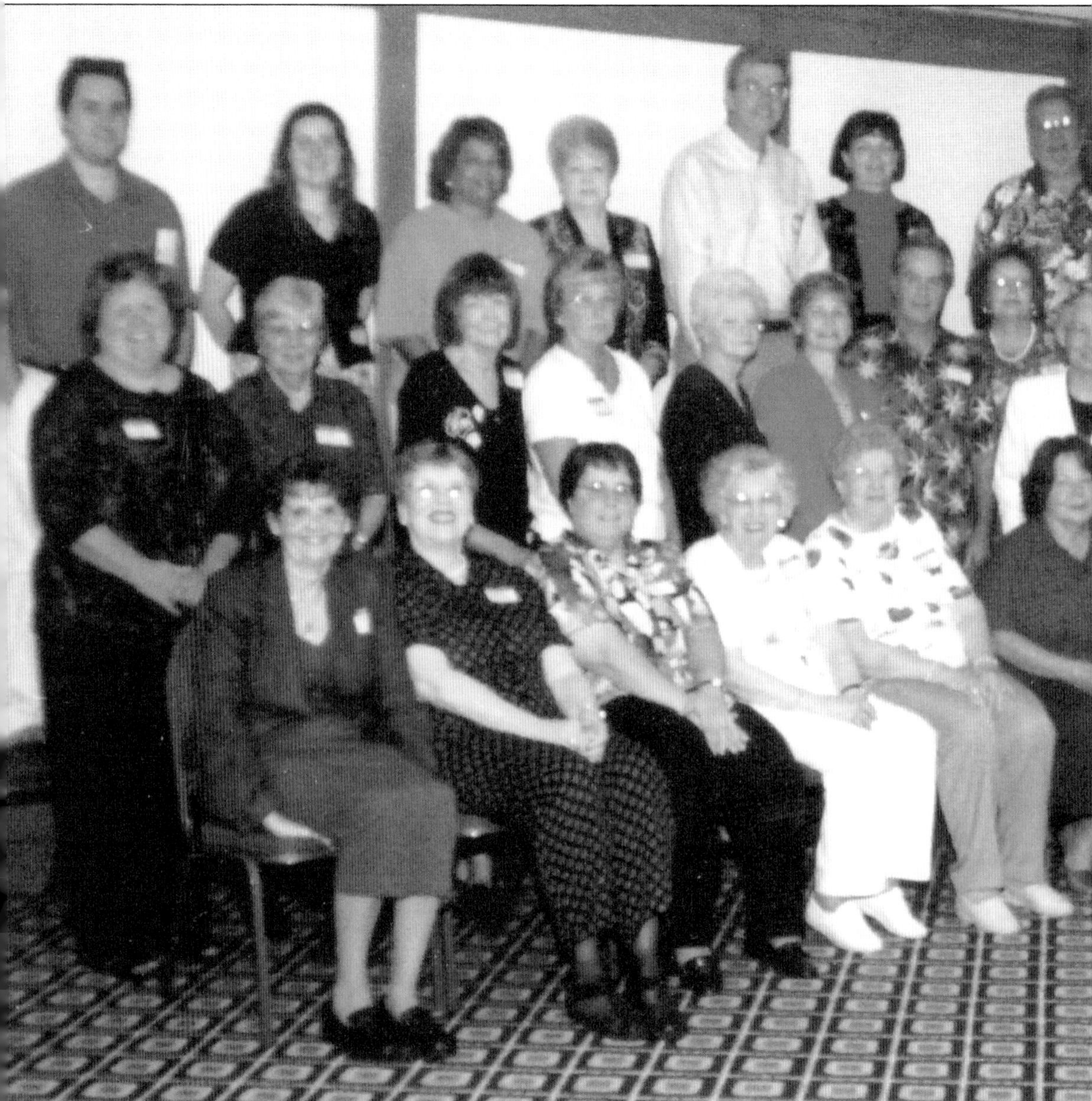

The Dixmont reunion, which is held on the last Friday of September on even years, is a celebration of former Dixmont employees. They are organized by Helen Wolf and usually are held at the Sewickley Country Inn, a local hotel and restaurant in Sewickley. The event has been a success for more than 20 years and typically ends with a group photograph. The event is booked for

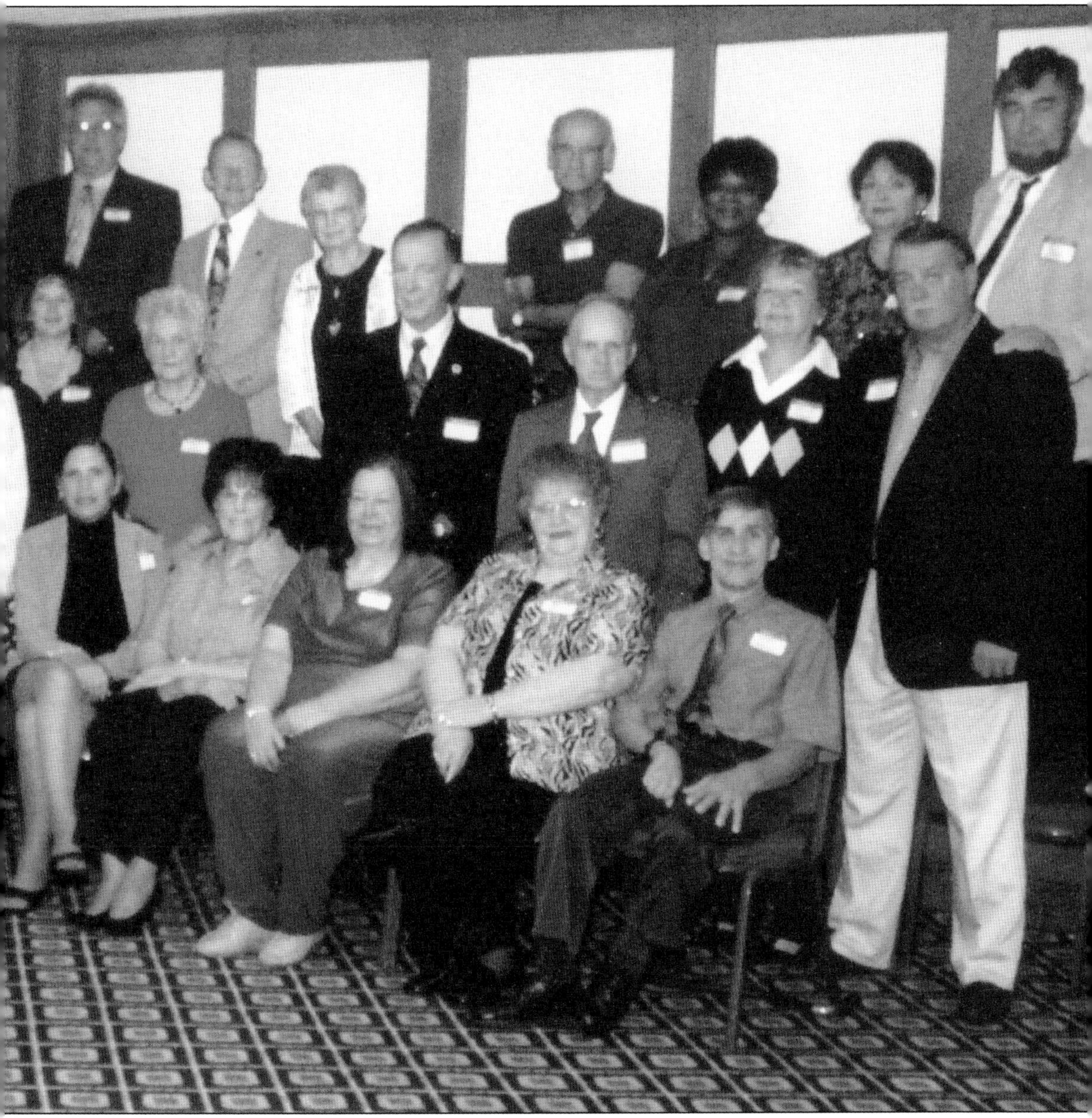

September 29, 2006. Jack Lennon typically emcees the event and employees reminisce, watch old films taken at Dixmont, look at photographs, and remember their friends who have passed away since the last reunion. (Courtesy Walter Sickles Photography.)

Consistent with our mission to preserve history on a local level, this book was printed in South Carolina on American-made paper and manufactured entirely in the United States. Products carrying the accredited Forest Stewardship Council (FSC) label are printed on 100 percent FSC-certified paper.